FITNESS, FATNESS ... and SEX FOREVER

FITNESS, FATNESS ... and SEX FOREVER

*A slightly off-color, politically incorrect,
adult tongue-in-cheek guide to improved physical
fitness, sexual prowess and stamina
(especially for the males)*

Jerry Moore

iUniverse, Inc.
New York Lincoln Shanghai

FITNESS, FATNESS ... and SEX FOREVER
A slightly off-color, politically incorrect, adult tongue-in-cheek guide to improved physical fitness, sexual prowess and stamina (especially for the males)

iUniverse books may be ordered through booksellers or by contacting:

iUniverse
2021 Pine Lake Road, Suite 100
Lincoln, NE 68512
www.iuniverse.com
1-800-Authors (1-800-288-4677)

You should not undertake any diet/exercise regimen recommended in this book before consulting your personal physician. Neither the author nor the publisher shall be responsible or liable for any loss or damage allegedly arising as a consequence of your use or application of any information or suggestions contained in this book.

This book is intended to help anyone who wants to get his or her body into shape, increase their sexual capabilities, live longer and love stronger without drastically changing their life or emptying their wallets in such pursuit. Since there are numerous books and articles available primarily for the female population, the material leans more towards the guys ... but, ladies, don't let this dissuade you. Everyone can benefit!

ISBN-13: 978-0-595-43370-4 (pbk)
ISBN-13: 978-0-595-87696-9 (ebk)
ISBN-10: 0-595-43370-7 (pbk)
ISBN-10: 0-595-87696-X (ebk)

Printed in the United States of America

CONTENTS

PREFACE

Most information regarding physical fitness and sex is written primarily for a female audience. A quick glance at the magazine racks in a leading national bookstore some time back gave quite substantial corroboration for this statement:

The Oprah Magazine displayed this heading on the cover:

> *LET'S TALK ABOUT SEX (Stuff you've never read about in a nice magazine like this)*

How about **Redbook**? Same rack, on the cover:

> *A LIFETIME OF HOT SEX. YES!*

Even more suggestive covers were displayed by recent issues of **COSMOPOLITAN**, such as:

> *THAT CERTAIN KIND OF SEX HE'S THINKING ABOUT 24/7*

> *HOT NEW SEX TRICK This Mind-Blowing, Box-Spring Breaking Technique Will Intensify <u>Everything</u> He Feels*

> *WHAT SEX IS LIKE FOR HIM And How to Enhance Every Single Thing He Feels*

Want a book on the subject? How about *THE GOOD GIRL'S GUIDE TO BAD GIRL SEX an indispensable guide to pleasure and seduction,* or *SUPER SEXUAL ORGASM,* both written by Barbara Keesling, Ph.D.

Women's magazines and books strongly imply that sex and fitness are very important in a ladies life. Is this something new—a sign of the times? Maybe not. A quick glance at the cover of a **Redbook** dated March 1992 has this heading:

WHY EXERCISE MAKES YOU BETTER IN BED.

It appears that not much changed over the years… sex is great, and being fit makes it that much better.

But, how about articles for men? Same magazine racks—one or two musclebuilders magazines—nothing regarding improving sexual activity on any covers.

This book, **FITNESS, FATNESS … and SEX FOREVER**, is designed to fill that void. Because of some "earthy, male-oriented language" it may seem a bit strong at times. Actually, the information in the book may benefit any and all who want to get their body into better condition, and put some *Real Life* into their sex life.

INTRODUCTION

No one in his or her right mind wants to be fat or unhealthy. Everyone wants to be physically attractive to at least one other person in this world. So, why are there so many out-of-shape, overweight, undersexed physical misfits dragging their tired asses around the land day in and day out? Diets don't help. Exercise programs are shelved as fast as they get started. Libidos peak, and then start a downward slide that doesn't terminate until the undertaker is summoned.

Middle age need not be the initial stage of long-term planning for the rocking chair and involuntary celibacy. Quite the contrary. The body is like a classic car. Abuse it and before long the local tow truck will be by to haul it to the scrap heap. Be smart. Restore it. Put every part back as close to original as possible. Rebuild that worn-out engine. Eliminate the rusty spots. Treat the whole machine with care and respect and reap the rewards. Few things in this world are as exciting as a fully restored '57 Chevy Bel Aire finished with ten coats of hand-buffed lacquer. The same can be said for a man or woman with a finely tuned physique and that unmistakable glow of health. The decision is yours.

If the only thing you exercise in a twenty-four hour day is your jaws and your bowels, you are going to put on weight. Don't blame it on God. God didn't make you gain weight. Don't blame it on your ex-mate. He or she may have done some really horrendous things, but making you gain weight wasn't one of them. Job stress didn't make you gain weight. The fry cook at the local greasy spoon didn't make you gain weight. Don't accuse the fast-food joints, either. Barring a serious medical, congenital or hereditary problem… you made you gain weight!

And for the skinny guys standing on the sidelines with a big smirk plastered on their faces … don't get too cocky. Just because you can look down and see your toes when you straddle a urinal does not necessarily indicate that you are in any better shape than your rotund counterparts. You don't have to be a lard-ass to be a physical misfit. These come in all shapes and sizes.

As we get farther and farther from the womb, our baby fat starts turning into muscle tissue. As we get closer and closer to our final reward, our muscle tissue dissolves or starts turning back to baby fat. It becomes imperative that we do something, anything, to hold off this onslaught by Father Time, Mother Nature and the Grim Reaper.

If you are one of the many who has already taken action in this battle for longevity, health and happiness—this is wonderful. You probably bounce out of bed every morning like a coiled spring, jog ten miles, pump iron for two hours, and dance around in your tutu to loud music for another half hour. More power to you. May you live to be a hundred, and consume a ton of oat bran and three thousand gallons of yogurt in the process!

But believe me it is not like that for the rest of the populace—the sloven majority. Getting out of bed in the morning can be a truly a major effort. The events that follow are not much better—slam dunk a greasy donut and a cup of strong black coffee, rush like hell to get to work on time, sit on your butt all day, bored stiff, come home, plop down in front of the tube with a six-pack of beer, stuff dinner down like there is no tomorrow, slither back to the couch, fart and burp until it is time to hit the sack, then start the process all over again.

Do these folks need a little change in life style? They sure as hell do.

The content and vernacular of this book primarily target the middle-aged American male. If you don't happen to fit into this narrow category, stick around anyway. Anyone, regardless of age, race, occupation, religion, or sexual orientation may benefit by absorbing and putting into practice many of the principles contained herein.

Before going any further, we should define middle age. In it's most simple formulation, it is the age attained approximately halfway between birth and death. Without the gift of clairvoyance, no one knows in advance at what point in time they will become an obituary, so a rough estimate can be deduced based on certain variables, such as life style, personal habits, family history and so on. Insurance companies come pretty close with their actuarial tables. For example, a non-smoking businessperson who exercises regularly and eats sensibly should live to be around eighty, and middle age would be somewhere around forty. On the other hand, an out-of-control party-animal who consumes a quart of hard liquor in one sitting, wipes out three packs of cigarettes a day, eats only food fried in animal fat, beds down every douche-bag bar-fly in town, and can't even spell the word exercise, may find middle age to be closer to his late teens.

By now, you may be thinking that the world needs another fitness book like you need another hole in your head. This may or may not be true. I do think that you will find this book quite a bit different that any other fitness book you may have read. And, on that subject, how many fitness books have you read from cover to cover? Come on now… be honest. Chances are, before you read this introduction you checked out the chapters on sex muscles. Right? There is also a good chance that there are some who are reading this book because, in reality, they have the sex drive of a crescent wrench, and are shaped like a beer can with arms and legs. Well, believe it or not, one can transform that mass of flesh they call a body into a reasonable facsimile of a physical specimen without a whole lot of effort. You don't have to dance around to ear-splitting music, dressed like Tinker Bell. You don't have to mortgage your home to pay for six months membership in the local health spa. And there is no need to spend eighty bucks on aerodynamically designed calfskin running shoes, or twice that much on custom designer sweats.

Would you believe that you can do almost everything in the privacy of your own home? There are even some very private exercises that you can do in church or standing in line at the bank or supermarket, or at your desk at work, without anyone being the wiser. What special equipment do you need? How about chairs, bathroom sink, a doorknob, grocery bags? Are there really exercises that can help, you know, with … sex? There sure are! Think about it for moment. Why should your private parts wear out any quicker than the other parts of your body? Things may slow down a little with time, but your equipment was designed to function until the last rites are read. Ask anyone who has worked in a home for the aged. You will invariably hear stories about horny old guys in their nineties with that familiar urge, chasing young seventy year old gals up and down the halls. And don't be fooled by some of these sweet innocent-looking little senior ladies … a knitting needle may not be the only solid object they have on their minds.

The sex-muscle exercises described in this book are simple, fun-to-do, and designed to awaken that power-packed sexual vigor you have lusted for in your most lurid, erotic dreams. Unfortunately, becoming fit and healthy requires more than just doing a few exercises. If you regularly slop down at the food trough like a barnyard pig, you will be a sure loser in the battle to bind the bulging buttocks. No need for alarm though—a tasteless, meatless, fatless, fun-less diet is not necessary—just some minor adjustments to your daily eating habits.

And, before you go out on the prowl to try out your newly acquired power-packed sexual vigor, you should be aware of the darker side of the world of lust. Nasty, deadly diseases are lurking around just waiting to get caught, and, without precautions, the chance of unexpected fatherhood and motherhood is also forever lurking.

You may be wondering who the heck is the author of this book, and what makes him such an expert. To begin with, he does not claim to be an expert. He was a successful college athlete, and during thirty-three years as a professional fire-fighter saw an unbelievable amount of self-induced misery and death—massive heart attacks in people much too young to deserve such a demise, bodies totally wasted by lung cancer and emphysema. A lot of these corpses would still be alive and kicking if they had not let their bodies go completely to hell.

And, sad to say, it doesn't look like things are going to improve too much in the future. For example, did you know that a large percentage of the high schools in the United states do not require their students to take physical education. Worse yet, in the schools that do require it, only half of the kids participate. Put these figures into your calculator, and you should discover that up to three-fourths of our offspring might well be sitting on their butts all day in school <u>and</u> at home. If this isn't bad enough their older counterparts don't seem to be doing much better. Reports from some airlines indicate that the average weight of passengers is going up. Not only does this add to fuel costs, some passengers are being required to pay for two seats. Disgraceful.

Incidentally, during his firefighting career the author incurred severe injuries to both his back and his neck, but is able to utilize the simple exercises in the book with no discomfort or strain. There are no guarantees that you will be able to turn those excess pounds of drooping flesh into massive pillars of rock-hard muscle tissue or svelte, eye-catching figures of beauty. But, if you wind up feeling better, looking better, and living and loving a little longer, then it should be worth the meager investment.

FITNESS

CHAPTER I

WHAT CAUSES THAT BULGE?

Most of us have a bulge here or there. Unfortunately, not the kind of bulge that one reads about in letters to the editor in Penthouse Magazine. To be blunt, too many of us bulge with unwanted fat. And, it shows. Unless you are really clever, there is no way to hide that excess pork with flattering clothing. Do you want muscle or blubber to be what's pushing your epidermis against those tight-fittin'-jeans? Men want MUSCLE! Raw, untamed, rippling layers of vibrant, twangy muscle tissue. Women want smooth, silky, lithe bodies that will make the rest of the sewing circle sick with envy and cause men to feel an instant surge in the central section of their southern hemisphere.

Let's take a minute and talk about muscles. Did you know that muscles have names? Everyone knows what biceps are. But how about the rest of the muscles? For example, the chest muscles are called pectorals, which is short for pectoralis majores. If you are into bodybuilding, you refer to them as pecs. How might this information be of any benefit to you? In many ways. For the guys, let us imagine that you suddenly spot a female with perfectly proportioned breasts. Instead of blurting out, "Wow, look at the set of knockers on that babe!" You might rephrase it as "My goodness, that attractive young woman has very well developed pectorals." You instantly establish yourself as a man of the world, with culture and breeding, instead of a horny, sexist pig.

If you actually plan to indulge in this, or any other program for physical self-improvement, you might find the following to be of some interest. You should, at least be familiar with a few of the basic muscles:

Muscle	Location	Slang or Short Name
Deltoids	Upper arm, by the shoulder	"Delts"
Trapezius	Between back of neck and shoulder	"Traps"
Latissimus Dorsi	Back, directly beneath shoulder	"Lats"
Gluteus Maximus	Cheeks of the derierre	"Glutes"
Abdominals	Stomach	"Abs"

Along the same lines, a few definitions come in handy, such as:

"Reps"   Short for repetitions. Means simply how many times you do something. This goes hand in hand with "sets."

"Sets"   Easiest to define this one by using it in a typical muscle-oriented sentence. "Like, man, I'm up to five sets of ten reps." To wit, he did whatever he was doing in five separate bunches of ten.

"Pump"   Akin to blowing up a balloon or tire. You do enough heavy "reps" to force large amounts of blood into selective areas of muscle tissue, ie: the biceps. They get huge. Caution, though. If you get enough of your muscles "pumped," other less-important areas of the body (such as the brain) may become blood deficient and starved for oxygen. Of, course this is a matter of personal priority.

"Definition"   As in well-defined. Obvious, visible boundaries or outlines that suddenly appear around muscles when one flexes said muscle or set of muscles. Can be impressive, but if overdone, can look weird.

"No Pain, No Gain"   A phrase borrowed from S & M enthusiasts, which means if it doesn't hurt, it isn't doing you a damn bit of good. Ignore this philosophy—it truly sucks.

Twitching

You should be aware that you have two different types of muscle tissue lying beneath your skin. First, there are the **slow-twitch** muscles. These fibers respond to slow, rhythmic movements such as aerobics, distance running (marathon runners reportedly may have up to 80% slow twitch fibers), brisk walking, swimming, bicycling, normal sex, and dancing. They don't grow much in size, but they build endurance. They require good old oxygen to function. The dark, or red meat in a chicken is made up of **slow twitch** muscle, with lots of blood vessels.

On the other side, we have muscles with **fast-twitch** fibers. Aggressive, calorie gobbling fat-fighters. They get their action from "resistance," i.e. weight lifting, isometrics (tension—muscle vs. muscle), push-ups, chin-ups, wrestling, uncontrolled wild sex and so on. World class sprinters may have up to 80% fast twitch muscle fibers. They give you strength and speed. These are the muscles that get <u>pumped</u>. Blood rushes to them like groupies to a rock concert. And when the blood hits, some of it sticks, and the muscles swell up and grow. They require something called glycogen, which the body produces from carbohydrates. What does it do? Basically, it turns to sugar (glucose) to provide energy as needed. On a chicken, the fast twitch muscles are the white meat.

Why is this information so important? Because, for a long time the aerobic lily-puts and the muscle beach aficionados were in competition, each claiming that their respective techniques for fitness were superior. Neutral researchers, with no particular axe to grind, discovered that some combination of both types of fitness technique should be beneficial for most average folks. Too much of one without some balance from the other could even be detrimental. Again, Mother Nature steps in … reportedly there are some **intermediate twitch fibers**, with a combination of both.

Whether we like it or not, as we approach our final reward, Mother Nature slowly strips us of some of our muscle mass. Even older runners can't slow her down completely by indulging in tons of running. That is, until they get some fast twitchers in action. Add a little resistance work and voila, Mother Nature is put on hold for at least a while. The bottom line? Try to combine some walking or swimming, cycling or whatever with your muscle building.

At this point, you may be pondering as to which kind of muscle fibers are found in the sex muscles? Theoretically it depends on how slow and rhythmic you are, and how much resistance you encounter when the action heats up—a little **slow twitch** here and some **fast twitch** there.

Chapter 2

Get In the Mood

Half of the battle in the quest for health and fitness lies in getting the lead out of our butts and getting started. Procrastination is the leading culprit. If there is a choice to do <u>anything</u> besides exercise, most of us will probably do <u>anything</u> instead. Exercise is not fun. Most of us sweat and stink when we do it. It's repetitive. It's boring. It's hard work, and it can cause an outbreak of the famous fungus twins … athlete's foot and jock itch.

That is why most of us burn out in short order with the tedium associated with the regimen of preparation necessary to actually performing any exercise. If you belong to one of those fancy exclusive gyms (now known as fitness centers, health clubs, spas, etc) you have to pack all your gear, shoes, shorts, sweats, towel, liniment, etc., drive through snow, sleet, hail, traffic and smog, search for a parking place, find a locker, and change clothes. By this time, your ass may be dragging and your temper is as short as your fuse. Finally, you find yourself standing in line simply for an opportunity to try out one of those computerized chrome-plated marvels of modern muscle-making technology.

Who needs all of this aggravation? Isn't it much more pleasant to find a nice quiet, secluded spot in the privacy of your own home? For example, the living room—there is usually adequate space, it's cooler, and one may even watch a little TV. If the Missus is having a bridge party or the minister over for tea, then the den, bedroom, garage or the basement should work just fine.

A strict routine is not necessary, but it is much easier if you try to do these things at the same time each day. Be reasonable. It isn't necessary to emulate the fervid jerks that spring out of the sack every morning at the first crack of daylight. You know the types—up and at 'em at 4 a.m. If you can fit it in, do it in the morning. After work suits some better. Others prefer to hit it in the evening, finish off with a nice shower, and then sleep like a baby.

Some experts claim that exercise just before a meal puts a damper on the appetite. Just after a meal is not a good idea, since the stomach is using a good portion of your blood for digestive purposes. Remember, we're not talking about hours of involvement here—many of us will spend more time daily in the bathroom than we will grinding out these few routines.

By now, you should have picked a setting, and some sort of consistent time in which to participate. Believe it or not your mental state plays an important role. You have to work on the right image. What is the right image? A lot of people are defeated even before they start because they have an identification problem. On a scale of one to ten, their view of their own self-worth doesn't even make the chart. Positive thinking makes a big difference.

If you aren't real proud of your present physique, let's say you have a hangover (ie: drooping skin and flesh that originates somewhere near the chest, picks up mass and momentum as it passes the stomach and continues southward until the full circumference of your belt is hidden from view), then an inexpensive sweat suit should fit the bill. If you plan to do some walking a pair of comfortable sneakers should be sufficient. It is likely that podiatrists and sports medicine experts would recommend top quality (very expensive) walking shoes. It's your call … some folks put thousands of miles on their old sneakers with no ill effects.

If you like freedom of movement, are not too ashamed of your "bod" and you are in the privacy of your own home you could try some of those dainty little undies that men are wearing these days. They resemble ladies bikini panties, with a functional flap in the front. They are pretty skimpy—some of them don't even have the functional flap, so before you can relieve yourself you have to pull them halfway to your knees. But, they come in all kinds of colors and designs, so what the hell, why not?

CHAPTER 3

MAKE IT HARDER

If you are a true slob, then you are an artist at avoiding work and effort in every facet of your existence. If you ever do any grocery shopping, which is highly unlikely, you would never carry a bag of groceries to your car, even if parked right next to the entrance (which it usually is).
The store pays a lot of money for grocery carts. They should be used. Right?

Once you are rooted into your couch or lounger, an 8.0 earthquake isn't going to move you. You wouldn't dream of getting up to fetch something for yourself. That's what God made teen-agers for, isn't it? The list could go on and on. Normally, you search for, and find, the easiest, most effortless method of doing anything and everything. But that's the old you. The **new** you does everything the hardest way possible:

> **Walk a block.** Barring inclement weather, park at least a block from your destination. No more battle to see who can get the closest parking space. A brisk walk to and from is good for you.

> **Offer to do the shopping.** If you have to carry a bag or two of groceries to your car, don't hug them against your body. Try this instead—hold them out in front of you as far as you can—the further the better. As you walk, you will feel tension in the muscles just above your crotch (the lower abdominals), your biceps, shoulders and back. You can even tighten your buns while you are walking. This could look a little strange, so if you have an audience, skip the bit with the buns. Use this method when you carry anything of moderate weight. Be sensible—if you try to carry something too heavy, you could be tempting a hernia.

Now for that couch or lounger. You don't have to give it up, but you can put it to good use. If you want something, even a beer, get it yourself. When you get up, don't slouch up. Get into a half-squat position, and then lift slowly, moving straight up. Feel the thighs coming to life. And, as long as you are on the couch or lounger, here is an easy abdominal hardener you can try. Lift your legs together until they are almost straight out in front of you, as near horizontal as possible. See how long you can keep them up there. Suck that stomach in while you're doing this one. Expend a little effort. You have nothing to lose but disgusting, slimy, greasy fat tissue.

Do it at your desk Once more, you have an opportunity to put your work environment to use. Think of ways to make easy tasks <u>hard</u>. For example, if you sit at a desk all day, then, once in a while:

> Reach under the desk in front of you with both hands. Try to lift the desk. Strain a bit—keep it going for a few seconds. Let a little blood curse through your veins. If you are really subtle you can do this exercise while engaged in a conversation with someone at another desk. This is one of the beautiful advantages of isometric type exercises ... you can perform some of them without anyone being aware.

> Push your chair away from the desk until your arms are straight. Then, place your palms flat on the top of the desk and pull yourself back in. This one could be a real bear if your chair doesn't have wheels.

> Lift and straighten your legs out in front of you under the desk. Hold them there a while. (See couch and lounger above. Same principle.)

> Put your palms next to you flat on the arms of the chair. Push yourself up until your arms are straight, and then ease back down. Do a few reps. (Remember "reps." See definitions.)

If your co-workers think you are getting a little strange, to hell with 'em. When you fly right by them on your way up the corporate ladder, they'll be standing in line waiting to kiss your fanny.

Do it anywhere When in college the author was on the Louisiana State University track team. His good friend, former All-American football star and Heisman Trophy winner Billy Cannon was also on the track team, as a sprinter and shot-putter. On a long, boring bus trip to a track meet in Florida, Cannon wanted to get in some exercise, so he decided to do a few bench presses on the back seat of the bus ... using the author as the barbell. After a set or two, Cannon finished by holding the author against the ceiling of the bus, with one hand and then the other. Anyone can be creative. Use your imagination. Even the greats do it.

CHAPTER 4

BEND OVER AND SUCK IT IN

If you turned to chapter expecting to find something having to do with licentious oral activities, you do have a dirty mind. But, as long as you are here, stick around. There are a couple of things that you can do at random that will help hold down mid-section expansion. You don't need a warm up period. It doesn't matter what time of day it is, where you are, what you are wearing, or even what you happen to be doing. And, they take very little conscious effort. One is simply bending over. The other is sucking in your gut. You don't necessarily do them in sequence or simultaneously (as implied by the title of the chapter). Let's take them one at a time.

Bend Over Bending over is just that. You can pretend that there is something of great interest on the floor, such as a piece of legal tender bearing a portrait of a long-deceased President. Is there a special way to bend down and pick up a dollar bill? The answer, of course, is no. There are probably as many ways to bend down, as there are people. A few, such as super-loose high hurdlers, can easily arch over and reach to the ground without bending their knees an inch. Show offs! Most people do a squat, as if there is an imaginary toilet beneath them. Then they reach down between their legs and get whatever it is they bent over to get. Others are more refined and genteel. They place one leg forward of the other, then dip, straight down without bending at all in the middle, and reach down alongside the forward leg and delicately pick up their prize. Even though this method seems a little sissified, it is probably the safest for those with a bad back.

Another easy method is a half squat with a half bend, resting one hand on a knee for a little support, and assurance for a return to an upright position. If some folks squat down too far, there is a good possibility that they will not make it back up. This method you might call a happy medium.

So, do what is the most comfortable, easiest, safest and most natural for you. In the process, you are working the muscles in your upper thighs, the abs, the hips, the lower back, and if you remember to tighten your cheeks when you straighten up, you can get your bun-muscles involved.

Again, a word of caution—bending over to pick up something that is not there looks a little odd, so doing it when you are alone is probably advisable.

You should do the bend-over fifteen or twenty times a day. This does not seem like such a big deal, but just for the hell of it, whip out your calculator and do some computing:
One year (365 days) times 20 bend-overs per day equals 7,300 bend-overs in a year.
Not too bad! By sheer numbers, this one little insignificant act might work wonders for your physique.

Suck it in Now that we are done bending over let's suck it in. Sucking in one's gut is a bit different than bending over. For one thing, if you are discreet, you can get away with a good suck-in just about anytime, anywhere, and even in the presence of other people.

There are three basic types of Suck-Ins:

> 1. To the Backbone Just as the name implies, the object is to attempt to suck in your belly so far that the navel touches the spine. Naturally, they don't really touch, but you will be surprised just how far back you can get. Notice that it is not necessary to hold your breath. That comes later.

> 2. Tighten up In this particular case, you don't really suck it in. You isolate and tighten just the gut muscles. Again, continue breathing as normal as possible under the circumstances, and hold the muscles as tight as you can for as long as you can. You can do this while standing, lying down or sitting. Don't forget that, when this is done in a sitting position, you are pretty close

to emulating the act of elimination. Watch you P's and Q's. Test yourself to see just how cool you are. Do this one while you are involved in a deep, philosophical discussion with someone. See if you can pull it off without being detected.

3. <u>The Big Breath</u> Now you stop breathing. Suck in the biggest breath that you can muster, and then hold it. Pack your lungs with air. Notice that when you do so, you automatically suck the tummy in. Feel around a little. Better yet, have your mate feel around a little and vice-versa. See how many muscle groups get into action when you take a massive gulp of ozone—both the upper and lower stomach muscles, the lower back, the rib cage, and again, if you really put your heart and soul into it, you might find a tight butt (your own).

Don't be an idiot and hold your breath until you turn blue, but hold it for twenty to thirty seconds if you can. Ocean divers, singers, and some athletes work at holding their breath for long periods of time—like four to five minutes. By the time they are done, their other body parts must be screaming for oxygen.

So that's it. Bend over and suck it in. It is a little weird, but the benefits should far outweigh the effort involved.

CHAPTER 5

FANTASTIC FOREPLAY

There are some things in this world that need a period of warming up before they work properly, such as conventional ovens, diesel engines, women ... and muscles. For ovens, the warm-up is known as "pre-heating." The primary purpose is to bring the interior of the oven up to a pre-designated temperature. For diesel engines (and the fairer sex) the object is basically the same—to get the engine heated up and lubricants dispersed to the necessary moving parts. For more detailed information, check the Cummins Diesel Manual or a copy of the *Joy of Sex*.

If you are in the kind of shape that one would suspect you are in, and you consume the type and quantity of foods that one would suspect you consume, you better check with your doctor before taking any drastic action such as exercise and sensible eating. Also, warn you spouse or other form of mate ... there may be a notable change in your appearance and your life style, which will undoubtedly arouse suspicion that you are secretly screwing around.

As for your muscles, if you haven't engaged in athletic activity since the eleventh grade, you may be in for a big surprise. With time and inactivity, your muscles, and, more importantly, the things to which they are attached, i.e. tendons and ligaments, lose elasticity and they get brittle. Have you ever tried to stretch a weathered, worn-out rubber band? "Snap-O." Your muscles are somewhat like that rubber band. Take them suddenly from complete rest to heavy exertion, and you may likely suffer uncomfortable consequences ... cramps, charley-horses, pulled muscles, or the "big daddy," torn ligaments. All of these afflictions are painful, ranging from a simple "ouch" all the way up to "holy shit."

Fortunately, our muscles respond favorably to pre-exercise conditioning, or warming up. If you fit into the classification of old fart (somewhere between 55 and 105, depending on who is judging you) then there is a good chance that you have experienced some degree of back trouble. Nothing that you will be doing involves heavy lifting, but it is always best to <u>ease</u> into any physical activity, especially if your spine can move in three directions at the same time. The large muscle mass located on the backside of the thigh, affectionately known as the "hamstring" is another one to watch closely. This is the large muscle that puts sprinters into severe anguish when it tears.

Basically, warming up means stretching and gradually increasing movement. You want to stretch everything you can. Move your body <u>slowly</u> in different directions, consciously trying to bring all necessary muscles into activity. Thrust the shoulders and elbows up and back, one at a time, then together. Touch your toes, twist the trunk a little, clockwise—then counter-clockwise. Bend to one side, then the other. Spread the legs, hands on knees, do a half squat, then bend forward. (Remember the Bend-Overs?)

If you can touch your toes without bending your knees ... great. Some really loose folks can actually put their heads between their knees and touch their elbows to the ground. Now that is really loose. If you haven't been able to touch your toes for 15 or 20 years, cheat a little.

Stretching Things

> <u>Hamstrings:</u> *Stand with the legs spread wide, straighten both legs and bend the upper torso forward as if trying to touch your nose to one knee. Slowly, cautiously, hold it for about 15 seconds. Then do the other side. Repeat 3 or 4 times.*

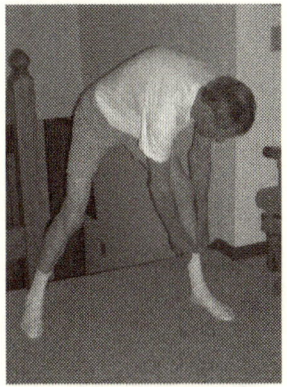 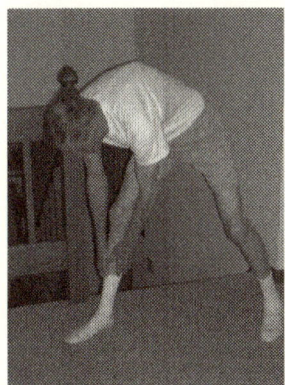

<u>Calves:</u> *(the lumps of muscle on the back side of shin bones) With your arms out in front of you, lean against a wall or door with one leg forward. Keep the back leg straight, foot flat on the floor as you lean further forward. When the calf muscle is tight, hold the position for several seconds. Switch legs and do the same routine.*

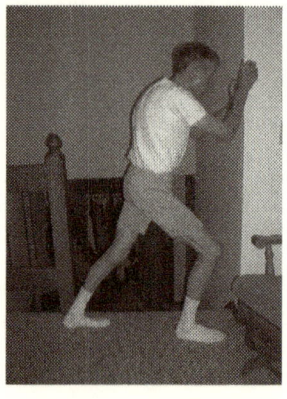 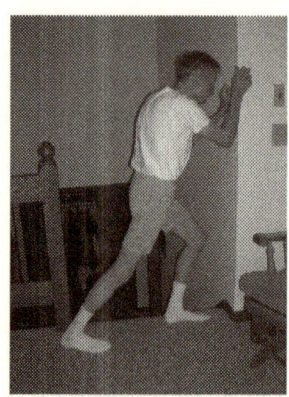

Continue this action, switching legs several times. When finished with this stretching, your body should be warmed up enough to get it on. If you are creative, you should be able to come up with some pretty outrageous stretching maneuvers for the rest of your body. Whatever it takes. Just get it all loose, and keep it all loose. After you finish working out, stretch things again. This gives your body a chance to get back to its normal sedentary condition.

CHAPTER 6

YA GOTTA HAVE HEART

No matter how you cut it, these exercises we are doing are not going to get your heart rate up significantly. The ones we have done so far, using resistance and tension, are supposed to build strength and activate the fast-twitch muscles to mobilize and grow in size. But, there are two parts to the health and fitness equation. To do the job completely, you have to get the blood rushing rapidly through the whole machine—make the ticker work a little harder. Cardio-vascular.

By now, some disenchantment may be surfacing. You expected to build a great body and all that other stuff in "just a few minutes a day." You have been at it for ten minutes already, you are tired, you are sweaty, and you want a beer. If you are inherently naive enough to believe that you are going to get that trashed body into shape in just ten minutes a day, you probably invested in ocean beachfront property in Nevada.

Be honest. Don't you feel better, more energetic and dynamic?

You have roughed it out this far. Hang in there, it can only get better.

Let's get the blood moving. How?

Jogging Of course, there is always … jogging It can be extremely beneficial. It can be done on the sidewalks or streets by your home, at the high school track, or on special trails that some localities provide. It does have some potential downsides: While shuffling along beside the highway, gasping for air, you may be filling your lungs with all of the residue contaminants of vehicular exhaust emissions: carbon monoxide, toxins, carcinogens and nasty elements not even classified as yet.

Your internal organs may get slammed against each other. Remember, these are fragile body parts—there is no factory warranty for replacement if they become damaged or dislodged.

You can become an object of ridicule. Your belly rolls and wiggles incessantly with every stride. Sweat seeps out of every pore on your body, reflecting sunlight off of the jiggling undulations of cellulite. Your face gets red as a beet. Little kids point at you and giggle. Older folks just stare in bewilderment. If the ladies are more than moderately endowed, it is often difficult to restrain the boobs.

Jogging in circles around a track can be worse. You may get morose from the monotony and boredom. Junior high school kids sneer with the mockery of youthful superiority as they zip by on the curves. Even so, if you are into it and enjoy jogging, ignore this satire and keep it up—it is definitely cardiovascular and one of the most popular forms of exercise.

Aerobics How about aerobics? If you have tried them and like them, you know that they can do the job. Some programs are wonderful, and highly effective. Some are not. Be selective.

Many of the programs are designed for the already super-fit. The instructor fires commands so fast that you find yourself three exercises behind in no time—and quickly pooped. If you can keep up with these sadists, you sure as hell don't need to read a book like this.

You have to dress weird. Tutus don't do anything for the masculine image, and those tights for the ladies look great on a size 3 frame, but for most forty-year-old mothers who have struggled through three pregnancies it may be a different story.

You are not your own person. You are being ordered around like a subservient cur. "Do this, do that, lift your legs, lower your butt, speed it up, slow it down."

Your ego can suffer as much as your tendons and ligaments. You can't keep up, even with the porkers, so you start to think something is wrong with you. You begin to think about what you gave up to do this stuff—the couch, TV ball games (or soap operas), beer and nachos, long naps. For some, it can really be discouraging. So, what are your alternatives?

Swimming This is a great all-around slow-twitch exercise. If you have a pool, or access to one, that is wonderful. There are even complete aqua-exercise programs available. Try the YMCA, or the high school, or the local park pool. A good half hour three or four times a week should get you going. Note: Sitting stark naked in a hot tub with magnum of champagne in one hand and your sweetie in the other does not qualify in this particular category (but don't let that deter you).

Bicycling You can peddle your ass all over town. If you don't think riding a bike can prime your pump, try a couple of long, gradual steep hills. Your thighs will throb like … well, they will really throb. This can be a real cardio-vascular experience. Needless to remind all: if you have been as sedentary as a beached whale for numerous years, start out slowly. One over-indulgent tour and you won't have to worry about cardio-vascular any more. Also, watch out for traffic, you might be taking your life in your hands.

Stationary Bike Maybe you prefer privacy. Maybe you can't break your addiction to the tube. No problem. Get a stationary bike. You can pick one up pretty cheap at a garage sale. (These things do seem to get repeatedly re-cycled.) Peddle away to your hearts content while you watch the ball game or favorite soap. You like to read? Rig up a book holder.

Bench Step The bench step has been around for a long time. A few years back it was suddenly "discovered" and received a lot of play in the fitness circuit. There is really not much to it, but it is a great way to get vascular activity. Find something solid, six to twelve inches in height that will hold your weight—like a short bench, stool, wooden box, a stair, etc. Step up onto the bench with one foot, lift your weight as you raise the other foot, and you wind up standing on the bench with both feet. Then step back down. That is all there is to it. You can begin with one foot for a few reps, then switch. Wonderful aerobic action.

Bounce, Bounce Many years ago, when the author was junior high school age, his brother Mike would spend at least an hour every day in the middle of their front room—bouncing. He would jump up and down on one foot three or four times, and then switch to the other foot … on and on, and on. He called them "jumping exercises" and told the author to do them too. Since he thought that his big brother could walk on water, he bounced and bounced too. It was one of the smartest things he ever did. Brother Mike, not quite six-feet in height, developed so much spring in his legs that he was one of the best high school high jumpers in the nation, leaping over 6 feet 5 inches. Very few high-schoolers could dunk a basketball back in the early 1950s. Mike could do one-hand or two-hand dunks. He almost ended his athletic career when he caught his elbow on the rim and nearly ripped the backboard off the wall. Damage done to ligaments when he tried to extend a long jump by folding his legs before landing did finish his career. The "jumping exercises" paid the author's way through college. Only five feet-eight inches in height, he was able to dunk, and the extra jumping ability helped him to do well enough in the pole vault to earn a full scholarship to LSU, set a school record, and win the Southeastern Conference title. Today, Mike's "jumping exercises" are very popular, have a fancy name, and the results have been tremendous increases in athletes jumping abilities. They are called Plyometrics and the concept has broadened to include "bounding, hopping and hurdling." Anyway, the "bouncing exercises" do work. So, definitely include them.

Walking Guess what? Walking is the greatest, easiest, and most accessible of all aerobic type exercises. You can get all of the benefits of jogging with less potential body tissue destruction. Lots of folks are into walking now. There are walking clubs and walking magazines. Walking trails are being opened almost everywhere. You can even walk all the way across the United States on trails. Put on some comfortable sneakers or walking shoes, grab a small radio or tape player with headphones, open your door and go. You should try for at least twenty minutes at a fairly brisk pace. If you cannot find a spare twenty minutes at one crack, some walking experts say that two or three brisk ten-minute walks are just as good. Don't just stroll. Give it a little gusto.

Will this cardio-vascular activation help you to live longer?

You bloody well better believe that it will.

CHAPTER 7

Get it On and Cheat Without Guilt

Doing it With Chairs

If you wanted to, you could put together a complete exercise program using just two chairs. It is said that O.J. Simpson wrote a book on using chairs and other such items for exercise, so it must not be too bad of an idea—he was a pretty good athlete in his earlier days. A couple of dinette type chairs will work for us here … sturdy, not too heavy, with short backs.

CHAIR CARRY

Facing the back of the chair grasp the sides approximately halfway up the back. Standing as erect as possible, try to keep your arms straight as you lift the chair upward in front of you. Hold this position as long as you can, then slowly return the chair to the floor. To move the chair from place to place, do so while the chair is still being held level with the floor.

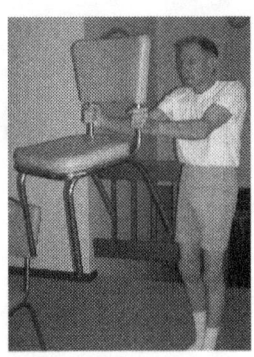

CHAIR AB LIFTS

Almost any firm chair can be used for Chair Ab Lifts. Sit in the chair with your hands holding the sides of the chair. Brace yourself as you attempt to lift your forelegs out straight in front of the chair. Hold this position as long as you can, then lower the legs back to the ground. Repeat this routine as many times as desired.

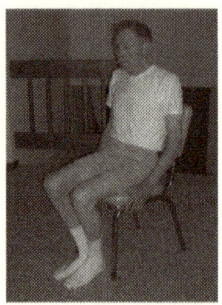 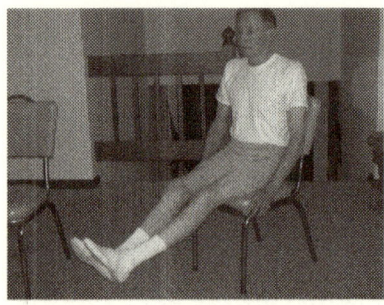

CHAIR PUSHUPS (single chair)

These are just like push-ups on the floor, except they are quite a bit easier. If you prefer to do them on the floor go for it. If not, read on.

Assume the position shown in the picture, facing the front of the chair, body straight and rigid. Adjust the angle until you feel comfortable. Keeping the body rigid, sink down as far as you can go, then push back up. See how easy. How many reps should you do? Do a few to see how they feel, then establish a number of reps

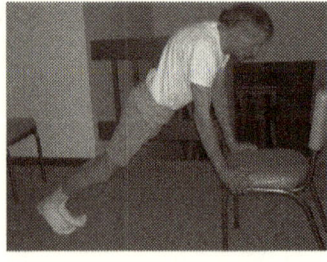 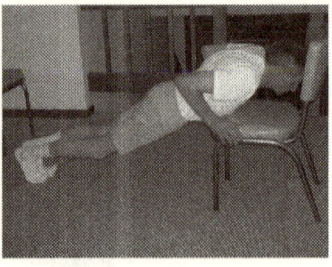

Don't get carried away and try to break an Olympic record. If you can't do any at all, don't despair—CHEAT.

CHEATIN' CHAIR PUSHUPS (single chair)

With one leg placed forward, pushups become a piece of cake. Switch legs half way through your set of reps. What have you accomplished up to this point? You have brought into action your triceps (the back of your upper arms), your chest, your back, and even the muscles around your ribs. Feel the surging blood rushing to feed that starving muscle tissue. You are on a roll.

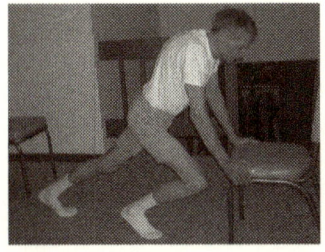 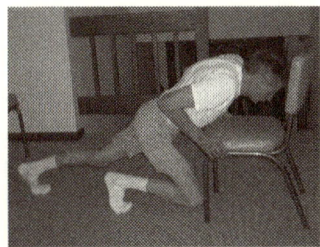

CHAIR PUSH UPS (two chairs)

Using two chairs gives you the advantage of dipping deeper, thereby getting more muscle mass involved. Place the chairs opposite each other a couple of inches farther apart than the width of your shoulders. Assume the same starting position as with the regular CHAIR PUSHUPS. Keep your body rigid, dip between the chairs as far down as possible, and then push back up. Feel that extra muscle action.

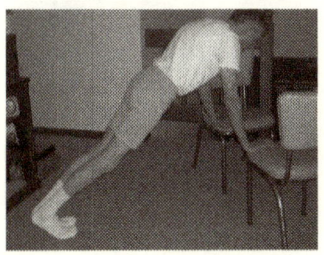 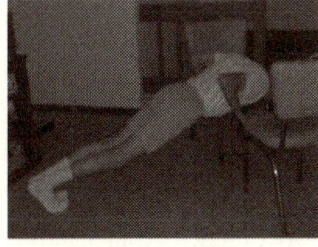

CHEATIN' CHAIR PUSH UPS (two chairs)

Use the same procedure as the single chair CHEATIN' CHAIR PUSH UPS above, so you will place one of your legs forward to relieve some of the weight. Do as many reps as feels comfortable.

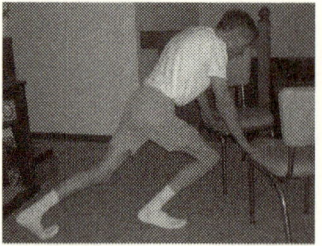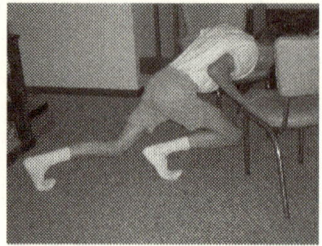

CHAIR CURLS (two hands)

For some reason, the biceps are the most basic indicator of muscularity. Some of the luckier folks can do one set of curls and their biceps blow up like helium party balloons. Others, like the author, are endowed with puny biceps and could pump all day with only a trace of noticeable swelling. Even so, curls are a must. Using both hands, stand behind the chair with your feet a few inches apart. Grab the chair uprights on each side just above the seat. Keep your arms straight. Lift slowly—keep your elbows close to your body, with your back straight. Pause. Let the chair down, also slowly. Do as many reps as comfortable.

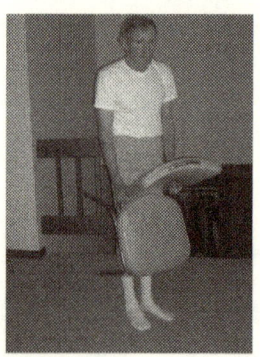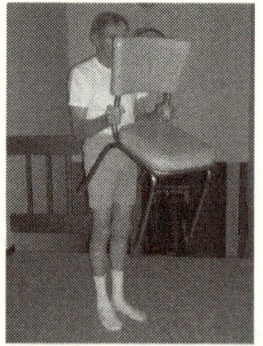

CHAIR CURLS (one hand)

If the chair is light enough to curl with one hand, the procedure is a little more complex. Approach the chair from the back. Spread your legs about 18 inches. Twist the chair so that one rear leg of the chair is between your legs. Grab the upright just above the seat cushion, getting it balanced as much as possible. Now, lifting it is no problem. Getting it back down requires a little caution. If you aren't careful, you might give yourself a whack in the juevos, and quickly lose interest in this whole program. Also, take it slow. Do as many reps as comfortable. Switch arms and repeat same procedures.

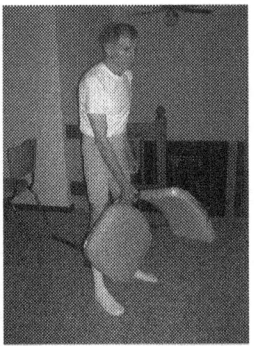 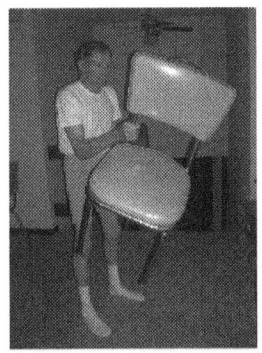

PUSH UP CHAIR SQUATS

Next, you can get your thighs involved while working on the triceps. Push up chair squats sounds rather dumb, but that is the best name that comes to mind for this routine.

Stand behind the chair with your legs, toes pointed out, about twelve inches apart. Put your arms down straight with the palms on the top of the back of the chair. Slowly start dropping down, keep the back straight. Spread your knees outward—like a ballet dancer. Go down far enough for your chest to be level with the top of the chair. Push back up, letting your arms do as much of the work as possible. As you reach the upright standing position, tighten your glutes (gluteus maximus, butt muscles). The more muscles you can involve, the better. You should be able to do at least a dozen of these.

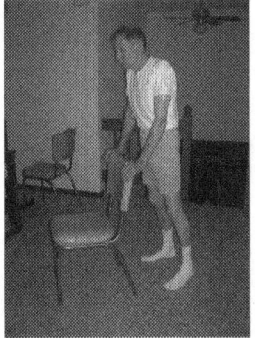 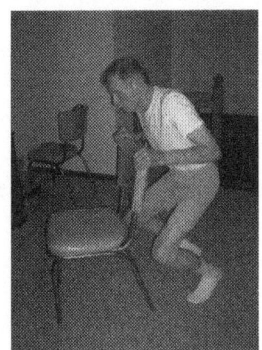

CHAIR DIPS

Place the chairs facing back to back, about the width of your shoulders. Stand between the chairs, arms straight down, palms on top of the chair backs. Take as much weight off of your legs as you can. Keep your back straight. Ease yourself down as low as you can comfortably, and then push yourself back up. Do as many reps as you can. Shoot for at least ten.

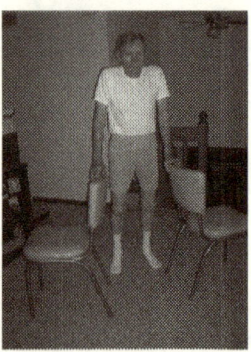 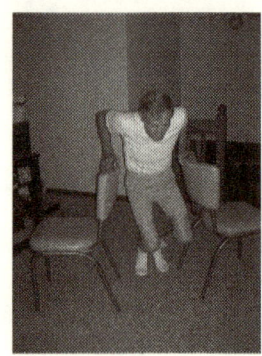

Motel, Hotel and Bathroom Routine

1. **Hotel or motel room** If the available chairs will work, you can perform the chair exercises, such as chair pushups, cheatin' chair pushups, chair curls, push up chair squats and chair dips

2. **In any bathroom** At home or in a hotel or motel, the following very simple set of exercises can be used, as shown in the illustrations.

RESISTANCE ARM CURLS

While standing straighten your right arm and place it an inch or so in front of your right thigh, hand formed in a fist. Cover the fist with the left hand and apply tension as you raise the right forearm in a curl movement. Continue to apply tension as the forearm moves back to its original position. Repeat the movements (reps) to complete a set of ten, then switch arms and repeat the exercise for a set of ten reps.

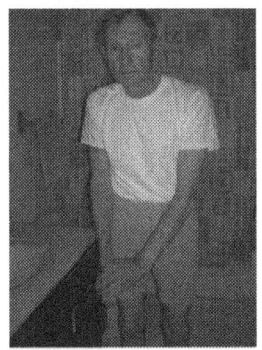 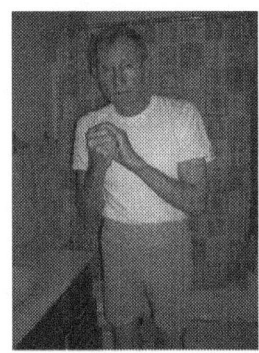

ONE ARM DIPS

Stand next to the edge of the sink, facing left. Place your right palm on the edge of the sink, and straighten your right arm. If necessary, stand on tiptoes, or bend your legs enough to straighten the right arm. Lower your body straight down as far as you can go, bending the right arm at the elbow. Reverse the action by pushing down with the right arm to raise your body to its original position. Repeat the movements (reps) to complete a set of ten, then switch arms so you will be facing the opposite direction and repeat the exercise for a set of ten reps.

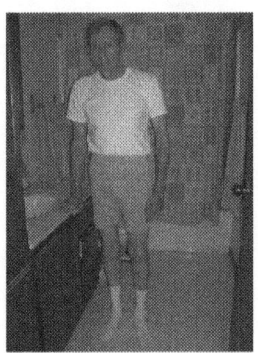 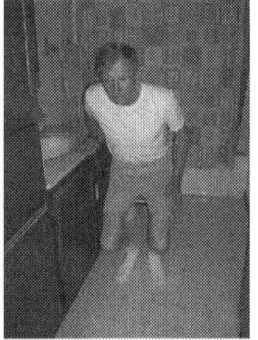

BICEP TENSION

Stand facing the sink so that with both arms straight, you can grasp the edge of the sink with both hands facing upward. Bend your arms slightly, then using only the biceps, attempt to lift the edge of the sink. Hold the tension as you count off approximately ten seconds (like thousand one…thousand two…etcetera, etcetera to thousand ten). Discontinue immediately if you hear creaking noises (from either your back or the sink}.

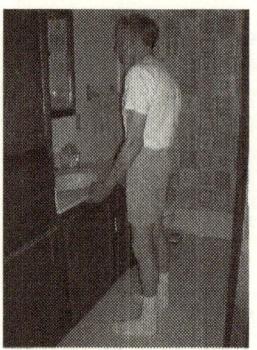

TRICEP TENSION

While standing facing the sink, turn your hands over so they are facing downward. Squat and lean forward slightly until the arms are bent close to 90 degrees. Using, as much as possible, just the triceps, push downward, holding tension, and again count off approximately ten seconds.

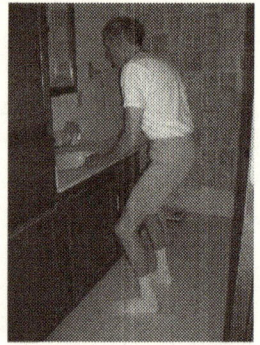

SINK SIDE PUSH-OUT

Lean over the front of the sink. With arms straight and hands balled into fists, center the fists near the top of both sides of the interior of the sink bowl. Again while counting off approximately ten seconds push outward against the sink sides with as much tension as you are able to muster.

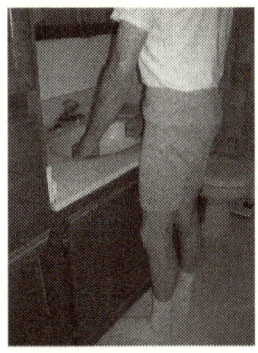

SINK TOP PULL-TOGETHER

Reach out with both hands along the front of the sink cabinet as far as possible. Grasp the edge of the sink with both hands and pull towards the middle with as much tension as possible. Once more, count off approximately ten seconds.

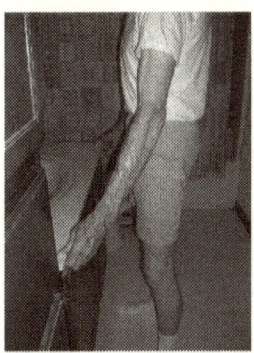

FORWARD SINK PUSH

Stand a few inches in front of the sink, arms extended straight down with fists formed. Move the arms forward until the fists contact the front of the sink or sink cabinet and apply tension against same. Hold tension again for approximately ten seconds.

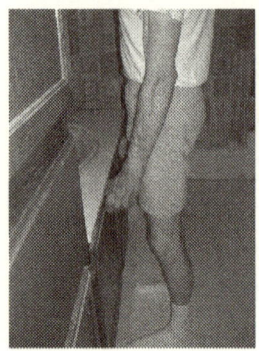

BACKWARD SINK PUSH

Standing a few inches in front of the sink or sink cabinet, extend your arms straight down with fists formed. Move the arms backward until the fists contact the surface of the sink or cabinet then apply tension against same. Hold tension for approximately ten seconds.

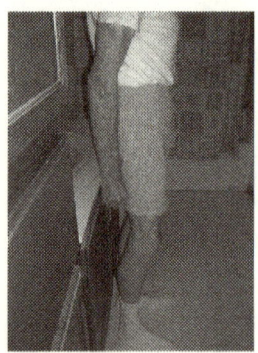

BACKWARD SINK LIFT

While still in the same position as for the BACKWARD SINK PUSH grasp the edge of the sink or any protruding surface, such as a drawer handle or facia. Using only the arms, do a lifting action to form tension and hold it for approximately ten seconds. Don't try to rip the drawer out of the cabinet—just use moderate tension.

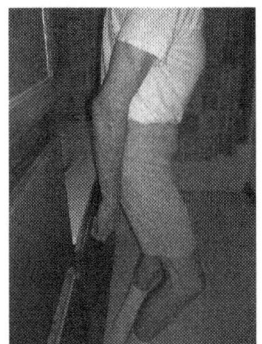

OVERHEAD WALL PUSH

Stand facing a wall or tall cabinet, arms extended almost straight up, balled fists together. Apply tension forward against the surface as if trying to push the wall down, keeping the body standing straight up. Hold it for around ten seconds.

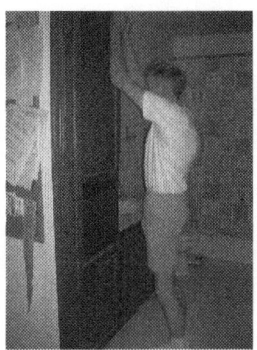

BACKWARD OVERHEAD WALL PUSH

Same action as the OVERHEAD WALL PUSH, except your backside will be facing the wall, and you bend your arms slightly and push backward against the wall. Once more, try it for about ten seconds.

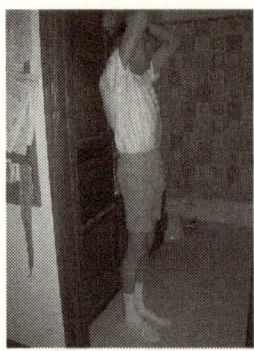

REGULAR SQUATS

Last routine. Standing a foot or so in front of the sink, facing either left or right, feet about 18 inches apart. Hold your balance by keeping a couple of fingers on the edge of the sink, and slowly do ten squats.

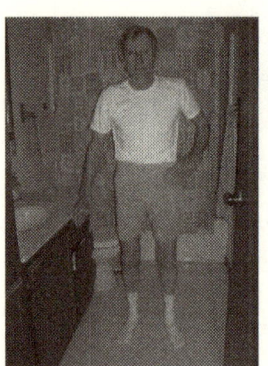 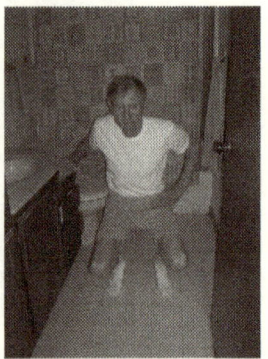

That is the complete **Doing it in the Bathroom** routine. See if you can fit it in before your shower or bath. It is relatively quick and doesn't require a lot of effort.

FATNESS

CHAPTER 8

WHAT GOES IN, DOESN'T ALWAYS COME OUT

The Engine The functioning processes of the human body can be compared to those of the automobile engine. Using this correlation in an overly simplified form, you can get a clear and understandable insight into the complex, mumbo-jumbo world of calories, cholesterol and fat. Please bear with the third grade type analogy, because you may be surprised by some of the revelations.

Fuel (food) enters the stomach. After a little anabolism and catabolism, the food is processed into useful and useless counterparts. The useful stuff is shuttled north into the blood stream. <u>Most</u> of the useless stuff is shuttled south into the dark, ugly caverns associated with waste removal. Note the use of the word "<u>most</u>" underlined. Not all of the unwanted ingredients that entered your body through your lips are filtered out in the metabolic processes ongoing in the depths of the stomach.

Once the fuel has entered the fuel line (blood stream), it journeys to the fuel pump (heart). In a car, oxygen makes its entrance through the carburetor. In the body, air comes in through the lungs, and the oxygen hitches a ride on some hemoglobin. From there it is parceled into the blood, headed for the heart through the pulmonary vein (for trivia buffs, the only vein in the body to transport oxygenated blood—all of the rest of your veins are trash collectors) sluggishly moving the fluid after it has dumped its oxygen and picked up a load of carbon dioxide (the gas that puts bubbles in your beer) and headed back to the lungs for excretion. In a day's time, you probably exhale enough carbon dioxide to carbonate a keg of Miller Lite.

At this point, the cells in the body become part of your engine. A sub-microscopic speck of food, or fuel, in the form of glucose, sneaks into a cell and gets next to the oxygen. They get cozy and form an explosive mixture (figuratively speaking). If you can picture this cell as a cylinder in an engine, a spark plug ignites the fuel/oxygen mixture and voila—energy. The cell does not have anything like a spark plug, but the same effect is generated by a process called *aerobic metabolism*. The energy that keeps the body alive has been produced.

Which cells get serviced first?

Those that need it the most. If you just finished a big meal, a good portion of the oxygenated blood makes a pit stop in your belly to get digestion out of the way. This flow of blood into an area is known as perfusion. Perfusion can be good, or it can be bad. The body builder's life revolves around getting as much blood as possible to perfuse to whichever muscle he or she is concentrating his or her resistance, ie: pumping. Conversely, someone in the middle of a severe MI (Myocardial Infarction—physicianese for a heart attack) would give anything to have more of that blood perfusing his or her clogged-up, starving, coronary arteries. Admittedly, this anatomical description won't get much credit as a thesis in human biology, but it will provide a base for what is to follow.

The fuel Are you confused by the steady bombardment of information thrown at us by health and nutrition experts regarding: cholesterol, fat, high density lipoprotein (HDL), low density lipoprotein (LDL), low calorie, high calorie, lite, low-fat, low-sugar and sugar free, soluble fiber, insoluble fiber, saturated fat, unsaturated fat, poly-unsaturated fat ... and the biggie at this particular point in time—trans fat, more scientifically known as ... trans fatty acid?

To get a grasp of this quagmire, we return to the auto/human body comparison. Assume that our car has a clear plastic, flexible fuel line. We can see what is going on inside of it, and compare it to our arteries. Unlike our food, we really don't have much choice of what fuel we put into our autos gas tank. We can be selective about brand and octane level, but are we really sure what it contains? No, we aren't. So, for illustration, let us assume that some quasi-terrorists got hired at all of our oil refineries. These workers are supposed to wrap little tiny doses of additives with a thin coating of a plastic-like material. These additives have to be wrapped so that a little of each is allowed to escape into the gasoline as it flows through the fuel line. One additive is "good" and one is "bad," but the bad is not all bad (actually, a little of it perks up performance of the engine) so it is OK if a little of it is allowed to escape.

The mission of our terrorists/workers is to screw with the amount of bad additive that is released into the fuel line. The thin coatings are tampered with, so over a period of time the excessive additive, which looks innocently like ear wax but eventually sets up like thick candle wax, builds up layers of deposits within the inside surface of the fuel line. If this is not bad enough, occasionally these creeps slip a wad of axle grease into some of the capsules. Most of these gunky little packages slip all the way though the system and get dumped into the interior of the engine as a sludge. A few spill bits of their load along the way.

Looking at the clear, flexible fuel line from the outside, we can see the build-up taking place inside. The once pliable tube has become brittle and rigid. Fuel flow is decreased. Only a small portion of fuel gets through to the fuel pump. The engine, struggling to function with less fuel has also become clogged with sludge and gunk. The scrap heap soon beckons.

Finally, it happens. A chunk of the crusty muck breaks loose and is carried though the lines by the flowing fuel. That is, until it comes to an encrusted area too large to get through. Suddenly, no more fuel gets through. The engine gasps, belches a cloud of bluish-black smoke, and shudders to a halt. CPR (carburetor panic rebuilding) is started immediately, but to no avail. The tow truck operator declares it to be a goner, and last rights are performed.

If you haven't guessed by now, the actors in the scenario should be obvious. No terrorists are involved ... the average American crams enough garbage into his or her mouth to eliminate any need for outside help from imaginary terrorists. Inside our bodies, the "good" additive is HDL, or high-density lipoprotein. Lipoprotein is the little capsules described above, the only difference being that the plastic-like shell is actually protein. It contains small bits of cholesterol, which are necessary for a lot of body functions. No problem.

The "bad" additive is LDL, low-density lipoprotein. It can carry large amounts of cholesterol, a little of which is also needed by the body, but unfortunately much of it gets dumped into the arteries. So, what happens? Just like in the fuel line, the crusty gunk that gets dumped builds up inside the arteries. It is referred to as plaque. You should be familiar with plaque. Think of the last time you had your teeth cleaned, and how the dentist chipped off your plaque build-up. Imagine something like that growing inside you blood vessels. Some of that axle grease traveling downstream eventually gets hooked onto the edges of plaque and can't break loose. Before too long a big grease-ball forms, waiting for a chance to get dislodged.

Oil and Grease Of course, it isn't axle grease floating through your blood. It is actually little fat globules, basically the same material that is left after you fry a greasy hamburger and let the residue get cold and solidify. What wasn't left in the pan settles somewhere else inside your body ... maybe on your chunky butt, slapped onto your thighs, or tucked away neatly into the folds of your belly fat. Nice stuff. It forms a basis for embolisms, clots, arteriosclerosis and other unpopular life-threatening conditions.

More bad news—some vegetable oils are as bad as animal fats. Pick up a carton of margarine in the super market. Try one with big, bold, bright colored wording that states:

"Made With 100% Vegetable Oil."

Check the label. Coconut oil and palm oil are two good examples of bad news. They are what are known as "saturated" oils, and may not be doing your system any good, although there is reportedly evidence though that <u>some</u> of the 86% saturated fat in coconut oil may actually be beneficial.

Now for some good news. Try the "other" kind of oils, the ones that contain "unsaturated fats." These come from various and sundry plants. Ever heard the terms mono-unsaturated or poly-unsaturated? How about like every day, in just about every other commercial on the tube. What do they mean? Mono means a little bit unsaturated (like peanut oil or olive oil). Poly means very unsaturated (like corn oil and safflower oil). They have one out that is supposed to be 100% free of everything. It is called canola oil. What is a canola? Who knows! It is made from rape seed, of the mustard family. Even though in its basic form it is so toxic that no insects will eat it, processed canola oil is about as good for you as it gets!

Is your spread hydrogenated? Sounds impressive. Maybe it means that the product is electronically infused with power-packed doses of hydrogen and oxygen. Not hardly. Hydrogenated means "hardened." Hardened oil or fat. Now we enter the world of **trans fat**. Try to imagine a major food producer putting something like *Made with pure hardened fat* on a label! That would be a really big seller.

Hydrogenation is necessary to firm up your margarine, etc. Even though it is made from pure vegetable oils, a hydrogenated product results in partially saturated fat. One thing is for certain … . trans fat sure as hell isn't going to help you harden up your you-know-what. The good news? At this point in time the FDA is requiring all manufacturers to put the presence of this nasty stuff on the label of contents.

What in the Hell is a Calorie? At last we come to something with which we should be familiar. The calorie. If you have ever dieted (and who hasn't), you have been beaten on the head with calories. Count them, avoid them at all costs, exercise to get rid of them, buy only items that say "low-calorie" on the label, etc. If you don't know what calories are, you must have ridden into town on the other pumpkin wagon. So … do you? Do you really know what calories are, and how they fit into this maze of nutritional nonsense? An Internet source says that 1 calorie = 4.18400 joules. What?? Try the dictionary. "A calorie is the amount of food necessary to produce one large calorie of energy." Wasn't that a lot of help? More definition. A large calorie is the amount of heat needed to raise the temperature of one gram of water one degree centigrade. Big deal!

Put the two together, and it appears that a calorie is the amount of food needed to generate enough heat to warm up a gram of water one degree C. It is absolutely amazing that someone was able to compute how many grams of Cheerios will cause a body to heat up a certain amount of water "x" number of degrees. For all intents and purposes, who really gives a damn? So, let's try a simpler definition.

A calorie is also a measurement of quantity. There are charts everywhere that will tell you how many calories in a mouth full of just about anything you want to take a mouthful of. An ounce of french fries will add 77 calories to your cause. Did you ever eat just one ounce of french fries? More like one ounce per bite. How about a piece of sugar-dripping, sucrose-saturated pecan pie? You're looking at 580 calories. This is definitely a more understandable definition.

But not entirely correct.

Not all calories are the same. Where that calorie came from has an influence on where it goes and how it will be used. Calories from a deep-fried French fry are going to wind up spending the night in a fat cell (and the next night, and the next, etc.) If all you eat is fat food, no matter how few calories you consume, most of them are going to join up with fat cells. Fat not only makes <u>you</u> fat, it hangs around in your stomach, slowing down the process of fuel production and waste disposal.

What about Protein and Carbohydrates? You want your calories to ride in on the "energy express." Your other two sources of calorie intake are protein and carbohydrates. Protein is what you get from lean red meat, chicken, fish, egg whites and so on. Carbohydrates are more from potatoes, bread, pasta, rice cereals and veggies.

Which group is the "energy express?"

Protein, right? Everywhere you look, it is high-protein this, high-protein that. People in poor underdeveloped nations are dying from lack of protein. It is extremely essential in battling malnutrition and many diseases. But, your body does not use it for producing energy. In fact, you don't want your body to be breaking down its protein for energy.

You want "carbos," Load up on the <u>right kinds</u> of carbohydrates. One-half to two-thirds of our calories should be packed in on carbos. These calories generate energy and break down fat. If you are a grease-eater, continuously assaulting your system with a diet that is 60 per-cent fat, all you have to do is reverse that figure with the one for carbohydrates, and you will soon be in the market for a smaller belt and a longer lease on that spot you occupy on this earth.

If you compare the major weight loss and diet programs operating today, you should discover that almost all of them recommend a ratio of roughly 50 or 60 percent carbohydrates, 20 to 25 percent protein, and yes, you do need some, 15 to 25 percent fat (unsaturated, right?). Muscle-rippling body builders might consume closer to two thirds carbos, one-fourth protein and only about one tenth fat intake. Lean and mean.

Who in the Heck eats Fiber? The next subject in the "mystery of munch" is fiber. There is always lots of disagreement as to which fiber product is on top of the polls at any particular time. This week it is oat bran, last week it was wheat bran, and now rice bran is becoming a strong contender. Of course, the old standbys ... apples, oranges, corn, beans and so on don't get the media attention that bran does, but they still get the job done.

What does fiber do?

Basically, fiber is just that … . fiber. If it is strong enough, we make rope out of it, like jute or hemp (the cannabis you weave, not smoke). The fiber meant for ingestion (but not digestion) comes in two forms—that which will dissolve in water (soluble) and, logically, that which won't dissolve in water (insoluble). Soluble fiber is supposed to dissolve into the system and kick ass on cholesterol. The insoluble fiber plows through the digestive tract like a plumber's power rooter, moving things along in the journey to exit and elimination.

Sprinkle on some poison Finally, there is salt—sodium chloride, also known as the mineral halite. Salt provides more useless trivia. Did you know that the two ingredients that combine to make ordinary table salt—sodium and chlorine—are each, separately, deadly poisons. What does salt do inside the human body that is so horrible? It holds water! That's it! It holds water—lots of water—like about fifty times its weight. If you consume too much salt, you are going to retain water. Water is heavy, and it bloats. Too much salt in the diet is extremely bad for those with hypertension. It skyrockets the blood pressure.

How much is too much?

Almost everything you eat contains a little salt in some form. One good juicy dill pickle has about half of your total daily-recommended requirement. Common sense helps. Popping potato chips all day long is not smart—salt-wise, fat-wise or cholesterol-wise. Even so, some salt is needed, without which you get cramps and other undesirable and uncomfortable conditions. A good rule of thumb: unless it is so bland that your tongue quivers in disgust, don't salt it.

That's it.

In a nutshell, we have covered the ins and outs of the relationship between cholesterol, calories, fat, carbohydrates, protein, fiber and salt. A picture begins to emerge. A little cholesterol is necessary, but too much is bad. The amount of calories consumed is important, but more important is the source of the calories (thumbs down on calories from fat, thumbs up for those from carbos and protein, especially the good carbos). Fiber is good for cholesterol bashing and smooth elimination, a little salt goes a long, long way, and **trans fat** is apparently the baddest shit on the whole planet.

Knowledge is power. If, by chance, the preceding information took seed and somehow remains lodged in the recesses of your subconscious, it could become an important weapon in your war against unchecked body spread. The author's experience with breakfast on-the-run is a prime example. For years, he dashed out the door with a cup of coffee in one hand, and in the other hand two pieces of toast or English muffin halves coated with peanut butter and jelly.

How do you know what portion of carbohydrates and calories a food contains? It is usually on the label. Remember all the stuff your momma told you about peanut butter ... "gives you energy, plus meat on your bones, listen to momma, momma knows." The author had implicit faith in the wisdom imparted by his dear sweet mother. Curiosity prompted him to take a look at the label on the side of a peanut butter jar.

<u>Serving Size</u>   2 Tablespoons (32 grams)

Calories	200	(A little high)
Calories from fat	140	(Surprise)
Protein	9gr	(Great)
Carbohydrates	6gr	(A Bit Low)
Total fat	16gr	(Fair)
Saturated Fat	3gr	(Bad News)
Trans Fat	0 gr	(Thank God)
Dietary fiber	2 gr	(Good News)
Sugars	3 gr	(So-So)
Cholesterol	0	(Wonderful)
Sodium	150 mg	(Pretty salty)

Even though seventy percent of the calories riding into the unsuspecting tummy were packed in fat globules, most of these are monounsaturated fat, which is good protection against heart disease. Since it also has a fair amount of protein and dietary fiber, an occasional dip into the old peanut butter jar is fine, although using natural peanut butter would eliminate any doubt.

How about a popping a couple of frozen waffles into the toaster, then a dab of "good" margarine and pure fruit jelly?

Serving size	1 waffle	
Calories	120	(Good Show)
Protein	3 grams	(Lost a little here)
Carbos	16 grams	(<u>Big</u> improvement)
Fat	5 grams	(Can live with it)
Sodium	250 mg	(Salty waffle)

It isn't necessary to walk the aisles of the supermarket with a clipboard and a hand-held high-tech multiple-memory calculator, comparing the nutritional value of every item of planned purchase. Shopping could become a full time occupation, as well as a real pain in the ass. But, there is sure no harm in comparing the ingredients of different brands of the products that you do plan to purchase.

Cholesterol, the Bottom Line

Some studies reportedly have shown that low cholesterol (under 160) may be as bad as high cholesterol (over 220), with the low cholesterol individual three times as likely to have a stroke and twice as likely to get cancer. Also, low cholesterol can be a factor in depression, suicide and anxiety. Isn't that a beaut? Work your ass off exercising and eating like a rabbit just to keep your pipes from clogging and your ticker ticking, only to find out that you are a prime candidate to croak from either a stroke or the big "C," or to have serious mental health problems.

Most interesting, and, most significantly, <u>those in the 160 to 220 range had the lowest death rate from all causes</u>).

That is something to think about.

CHAPTER 9

EAT IT, BABY

Now a most critical question surfaces … do you have to follow a "diet?" Webster's New World Dictionary should be sufficient motivation to cause anyone to avoid dieting, ie: "a regimen of special or limited food and drink, chosen or prescribed for health or to gain or lose weight." The key words are "regimen" and "limited food and drink." A best, this is somewhat discouraging.

Nothing has made more of an impression regarding diets and fat than a commercial that a well-known TV fitness guru did quite a few years back. He held up a one-pound hunk of greasy, ugly, dripping fat that was freshly cut from a side of beef. All that the viewer had to do was imagine twenty or thirty, or more, hunks of that slimy mess spread throughout his or her body. That, in itself, should have been enough to scare the holy crap out of the most avid cholesterol junkie.

Experts are all over the place with obscure theories about obesity and weight loss. Some claim that being fat is as much inherited as hair color, height, etcetera … and all of the diets in the world won't help. That is a very pessimistic outlook. Other experts write books about their own wonderful programs. Special diets, yoga, fasting, liposuction, tummy-tucks, jaw wiring, enemas, stomach stapling, and stomach by-pass—you name it, and you can bet that someone has tried it. Isn't it amazing to what extremes the human animal will go to shed flesh?

"It"

At one time some obscure researcher unearthed a startling revelation. You do not have complete control over your body weight. You are at the mercy of a little computer-like watchdog located somewhere inside you body …

no one is sure where the sneaky little son-of-a-bitch hides or resides. Anyway, "**It**" monitors everything about your body—what you eat, where the food goes, how many fat cells you have, how many muscle cells, etc. Without your advice or consent, "**It**" establishes a sort of personal thing called a *Set Point*. For adults your *Set Point* turns out to be pretty much your average weight. So, no matter how much you weigh, if you go about your business and don't rock the boat, over the years, your *Set Point* might remain fairly constant, but still is controlled by "**It**."

So, one day you wake up feeling like crap. You finally admit to yourself that you are a fat slob, and you are damned well going to do something about it. Call your doctor? Naw. Too easy. And what the hell does he know anyway—he or she is probably fatter than you are. So, you run right out and buy the latest, up-to-date-guaranteed-to-lose-50-pounds-in-ten-days-diet-book, (or your money cheerfully refunded). And, sure as heck, after ten days of eating some really weird shit, the needle on your scales agrees … fifty pounds of you have mysteriously disappeared. Where did it go? No one knows. It just went. Anyhow, in the process, you have really pissed "**It**" off. "**It**" does not want you fifty pounds lighter. "**It**" wants you right back where you were. In fact, in a little fit of vengeance, "**It**" will start screwing with your system. First off, "**It**" has quasi-magical powers that start showing up. How? "**It**" swaps fat for muscle tissue when you lose weight. Then, slowly but surely, over time, the pounds will come creeping back, and you wind up either at your original set point, or, quite possibly, even a little higher. And, your muscles mass may have dwindled proportionally in the process.

Not only did the latest so-called diet not work, you may wind up heavier than before, with more fat, less muscle, and in worse shape. This phenomenon is ungraciously referred to as the dreaded **yo-yo** effect. Maybe some experts who claim that being fat is an inherited trait are right, and the effort is all a waste. Right? Wrong!

You can beat "**It**." But, this is not an easy task. You have to fool the sneaky little bastard. We are all born with a certain number of fat cells, and although you can increase the number, you can't lose any of them. Even after liposuction, "**It**" can supposedly reproduce fat cells back to their original number—like a wacko scientist in a 1950s "B" science fiction movie. So, you see what you are up against.

But, even if you can't reduce the number of fat cells, you can shrink them. Not too fast, though. "**It**" goes nuts. Instead of dropping that fifty pounds in ten days, how about something more realistic? Like, one or two years. Since "**It**" spends most of its 24 hour day in the equivalent of watching soap operas (sort of brain dead), a very gradual decrease in the set point can easily go undetected.

Great, you say. But, that ten-day diet fiasco was a major bummer. If you <u>ever</u> try to lose weight again, you are going to set the ground rules. There is no way on God's earth that you are going to give up your meat and potatoes for pissy little portions of tofu and endive. As any enlightened teenager would say—"lighten up, Dude! Radical action is totally unnecessary." A few minor changes in your food intake habits can make a world of difference over a period of time. How about some suggestions:

> <u>If you insist on pigging out at one meal, do it at breakfast.</u> Some people even eat two small breakfasts and then skip lunch. Put this together with a reasonable dinner and you're already ahead. Remember—reasonable. If you gorge your guts at night, everything sits on the bottom of your belly like a huge hairball.

> <u>Try cereals</u> You don't have to use that super-bran jazz loaded with insoluble fiber. You remember what that stuff might do. Most of the old standards are still around and they work great. One of the major cereal makers has a suggested program to lose ten pounds by eating two meals a day consisting of their cereal with a measured amount of milk and a portion of fruit cup.

> <u>Potatoes are not necessarily fattening.</u> It is the carton of sour cream and the cube of butter you smear on them that hangs around after everything else has long been eliminated. Instead, be a little creative. Use reduced-fat butter. Sprinkle on some chives. And, maybe add a little picante sauce. Even plain non-fat yogurt. It won't kill you.

> <u>Go for loins</u> If you can't give up your macho-man red meat for chicken or turkey, then spend an extra buck or two for the leanest piece you can find—try "loins," like beef tenderloin. When you look at tempting steaks with hunks of fat surrounding the meat, remember the TV fitness guru's commercials. Enjoy some protein in its place.

> <u>Veggies</u> Still rebelling against your mother, aren't you? No way around it, dark green veggies are good for you (excluding the olive in your martini). So are the yellow ones ... especially if they are steamed. The more the merrier. Put the gooey cheese sauce back in the fridge. Ditto for the hol-

landaise. Instead, give Parmesan cheese a try, or soy sauce. Don't forget salt-free seasonings such as Mrs. Dash or Cajun Seasoning. Be creative!

Fruits Actually, they taste pretty good. When you get the munchies, eat some grapes, or apple slices. You can buy exotic fruits in your local grocery store these days, with undocumented aphrodisiac qualities—like cherimoyas, mangos, minneolas and clementines. Give them a try—they might even put some extra lead in your pencil.

One real hot item is fish Not only good for the waist line, fish reportedly has special oils that help clean your pipes. Remember though, fish does not have to be fried in two inches of 30 WT oil to taste good. Broil it, barbecue it, or bake it. Don't forget the Omega3—salmon, sardines and tuna are high in omega3 fats. These are fats that prolong life and reduce the aging process as well as expedite weight loss. Use a trans fat-free butter spread—it won't kill you.

Eat some pasta Or, how about rice? Some athletes, especially distance runners, eat huge quantities of pasta a few days or so before a competition. It is called carbo-loading (something to do with complex carbohydrates). Try whole-wheat pastas and brown rice. Much more nutritional bang for the buck. Be sensible though. You can't carbo-load every other night, then sit around on your lazy ass all day long.

Believe it or not, your greatest fat-smasher could be water Drink lots and lots of it. Externally, your body may look pretty clean, but, inside, it is a cesspool. Bacteria, toxins, chemicals, hordes of waste products abound everywhere. You are like a giant toilet. So, what do you do? You flush it. At least eight 8-ounce glasses a day. This does all kinds of good things. Almost all of the bad actors mentioned above get a one-way ticket to the city sewer system. And if you take a good slug before a meal, it might put a damper on that ravenous appetite. It helps burn off fat, expedites waste elimination, promotes healthy skin, helps fight off tummy aches and colds. Urine color tells tales. Real dark may indicate too little water intake. Key factor … the closer to clear the better.

There is one final little gimmick that you might try Fill your plate with your usual portion of food. Then put half of each item back You won't miss it. You have decreased your intake by 50% and it all helps in the bloody battle against the insidious "It."

Chapter 10

Heavy Metal

I believe it was Mac Davis in the movie *Rhinestone Cowboy* who referred to a female counterpart as the gal who could "suck the chrome off of a trailer hitch." Well would you believe that, with new findings in the world of vitamins and nutrition, this woman was way ahead of her time. Ingesting chrome is one of the "in" things. When this great discovery hit the news a few years back, <u>chromium</u> was touted as <u>the</u> great muscle builder, fat fighter and heart helper.

What does it do?

It has to do with insulin, a very important hormone that helps control blood sugar in our bodies. Let your mind wander back to the grand finale in energy production that takes place in your cells when the fuel (glucose) combines with oxygen and power surges through your body. Without insulin, the glucose couldn't get into the cell, and your whole system would be in a world of hurt. In addition to controlling blood sugar, insulin affects cholesterol formation, body weight (could this be "It?"), muscle mass, and a bunch of other things related to metabolism, such as slowing the loss of calcium, which may help women slow bone loss after menopause.

Without chromium, insulin can't do its thing. Obviously, chromium is important stuff. Some jocks and body builders are into chrome in a heavy way. Health food stores have all kinds of chromium supplements. Some sources can be found at your grocery store, such as calves liver, wheat germ, various cheeses and brewers yeast. Naturally, there is controversy over which type is the best, and there are some possible downsides ... high levels might be associated with glaucoma.

If you plan to give chromium a try, check with someone who is knowledgeable about the subject, such as nutritionists, medical researchers, and health food distributors.

Zinc is another hot metal (nutritionally speaking.) It helps the immune system do whatever it does, and breaks down food in the body for growth. Get this! The biggest user of zinc in a man's body is our old buddy, the prostate gland. What it does with all that zinc is anyone's guess, but if it doesn't get enough, you can imagine the consequences. The subject of metals that your body needs brings up a question. What about taking too much vitamins, minerals and all of those supplements we see advertised just about everywhere we look? The answer is debatable. It seems like a continuous running battle—some health food practitioners and fitness experts claim that you should take them by the handful, while a portion of the medical community insists that most are almost useless and possibly harmful if taken excessively.

Surely, at one time or another, you have flipped on the TV and found yourself facing a stern, somber-looking MD with clipboard in hand. He addresses the microphone—then in a voice so deep that you are sure he tucks his nuts into his socks, he sets the record straight. "If you eat a well-balanced diet, you do not need vitamin supplements." Well, Doc, we have already seen that the so-called average diet in the U.S. truly sucks, so whom can we believe?

The truth is, some extra vitamins and minerals are probably needed by all of us. Others are questionable—too much of some can be worse than not enough. What is a body to do?

How about a personal vitamin program? Here is one that is pretty basic:

> Megavitamins—Nothing fancy. Actually, a generic brand from a local supermarket may suffice. The author picked a particular one because the pills are not quite so big. This means that they are less likely to get stuck in the throat and leave that horrible "vitamin" taste in the mouth.

> Vitamin E—Take these in moderation. A cohort once confided that he would take a bunch before getting it on, and it gave him a little extra endurance with the old stiffy, and he said he could last for hours. Some say that 99% of sexual performance is in the mind, so, whatever gives you that extra edge, especially now with Viagra and all of its cousins. A

point of interest—some scientific studies also have shown that vitamin E may cut the risk of heart attack.

Vitamin C—The author is a firm believer in Dr. Linus Pauling. Before Pauling made his astounding findings with Vitamin C aiding in fighting colds and sore throats the author would invariably spend two full weeks laid up—at least twice a year—in total misery, with a boiling fever and massively swollen tonsils. No more. Now, when that familiar grating tickle in the throat begins, he jumps right on the "C's" ... four 500 mg pills every two hours and an occasional 400 mg Echinacea, until the tickle disappears. The results? No swollen tonsils in more than thirty years, and no colds or flu lasting for more than two days.

Calcium—Usually prescribed for women, but if you guys have lousy posture, and find that you may be a candidate for early Osteoporosis, try a little calcium. As a bonus it also makes for a healthy prostate, which helps with a responsive "Roger." Vitamin D is also reported to aid in preventing Osteoporosis.

Zinc—Oh, yes. As discussed earlier, zinc is one of those supplements that you have to watch carefully. Too much can be not so good, so to be one safe side, use the minimum recommended dose. But don't forget this one. Viva la prostate, and eat lots of pumpkin seeds and oysters.

CHAPTER 11

GET IT TOGETHER

Up to this point, everything seems pretty cut and dried. In review, we find that:

1. You need to exercise your fast-twitch muscles with some kind of resistance … such as the exercises in this book, weight lifting, push-ups, chin-ups, wrestling, screaming-hollering ceiling-bouncing sex, etc. This type of muscle fiber uses blood like a MASH unit and, in the process, burns up calories en masse.

2. You balance out your muscle work by some heart-pumping, oxygen-generating slow-twitch action: walking, swimming, climbing stairs, jogging, aerobics, riding a bike, normal sex, etc.

3. You have a general idea of the components and composition of what you put into your stomach each day, ie: protein, carbohydrates, fat, and the associated stuff—namely calories, HDL, LDL, cholesterol, saturated and unsaturated oil, vegetable oil, hydrogenated oil, plaque, soluble and insoluble fiber, and glucose. Come to think of it, you may know more about this subject than a lot of the so-called experts.

4. You are familiar with what happens when food hits your stomach, and

5. You have some inkling of what your body does with it after it passes through your stomach.

Basically, you should, by now, know pretty much what you should or should not put there in the first place. In the last chapter, you should have concluded that,

with minor deviations in your food consumption habits, which involve no dra-
conian diet measures, you can bring your self-destructive life-style to a slowly
grinding halt. In the process, you should easily reverse the supposedly irreversible,
and start your body on a non-stop journey down the path of re-shaping, molding
it into a thing of beautiful self-pride. Like a tree trimmer molds the shape of a tree.

This does not mean that your life should be totally devoid of its most basic pleas-
ures. Every once in while, we tend to deviate ... revert back to our previous, less
healthy ways. But, just temporarily. Which brings up a very interesting question.

Why do we love fat foods in the first place?

Probably because they taste so darn good. Visualizing a super-juicy taco from a
Jack-In-The-Box fast food restaurant can give one a nutritional high. You start sali-
vating like a Pavlovian dog, imagining that wonderful grease-filled mixture of juices
and sauces running down your chin. We all need an occasional bit of depravity and
harmless sin in our lives. As long as we keep up the exercises and sensible eating
habits (and keep the depravity and harmless sin down to a minimum) ... there
should be no problem. In the course of this quest for fitness and knowledge, some
surprises did leap out and make their presence be known, such as:

> Mayonnaise: For some reason, many folks have a distorted image of its
> composition and food value. Checking the label today, it doesn't seem so
> bad. Things like fat, cholesterol and sodium are judged by percent of
> daily value (DV) based on a 2000 calorie diet. Using a serving size of one
> tablespoon (13 grams) of mayo would only be 15% of your DV. Doesn't
> sound too bad. But, 10 of the 13 grams are fat, and all of the 90 calories
> in the serving come from that 10 grams of fat. Fortunately, only 1.5
> grams are saturated fat. Back in the early 1990's for the heck of it the
> author checked the label of a mayonnaise jar. Different system then ...
>
> protein 0%, carbohydrates 0%, fat 99%....

Ninety-nine percent ratio of fat? That's almost like reaching into the
intestines of a cow, grabbing a handful of stuff and mixing it with some
white food coloring. Calories? Humongous numbers. Lots of egg yolk
involved. Guess what? Artificial mayo tastes nearly enough like the real
stuff for any difference in taste to be inconsequential. Best of all, it is
loaded with protein and carbos, and almost no fat. Don't worry about
angering the manufacturers because you stopped buying the real stuff.

The same companies make the artificial stuff. Hedging their bets. There is also mayonnaise made with Canola Oil, no **trans fats**, very low in saturated fat. Keep in mind that the fat free and light mayos usually contain sugar, a reason why they are so palatable. If you really want the mayonnaise, a half-teaspoon will go a long way on a sandwich.

Phony fat: Chemists have produced honest-to-God imitation Fat. Duplicated the real thing. But it really is not fat—at least, not nutritionally. Supposedly, you can't tell it from the real thing, and it is almost totally real fat free. Pig out to the max, and don't wind up wearing it. This discovery should rate right up there with the cotton gin and penicillin. However, these phony fats, supposedly, have been known to give one a strong case of diarrhea.

Sugar: This is one of the biggies, and it has hardly been touched on. If you are sharp, you may have noticed that, in the nutritional breakdown on food labels, there is no mention of the amount of sugar in a product. It is there all right. It is disguised, as you will see later. Sugar has no nutritional value. Lots of calories, but no food value. Move your eyes a little to the right on the label, to the list of contents. You will find it mentioned. It may say simply "sugar," or it may show up as one or more of its' aliases: dextrose, sucrose, corn syrup, etc. Doesn't matter too much what form it comes in—once it gets to your stomach, it is, for all intents and purposes, just sugar.

Sugar is a "simple" carbohydrate. Other carbos, like pasta and potatoes, are "complex" carbohydrates. Probably, because, after they go through all kinds of gyrations and machinations in your stomach, involving starches and other chemical constituents, they break down into—sugar. Definitely not the kind of sugar that you put in your coffee in the morning. They break down into the kind that your body uses in the little engine cylinders (cells) to form energy. (Remember glucose?) Glucose we need, in a big way. Remember the ideal ration of protein-carbo-fat? Something in the order of 50-60% carbos. Well, since sugar is actually a "simple" carbohydrate, it can be listed on the food label under carbohydrates.

Some time back the author checked the back of a "Butterfinger" candy bar, and read the stats:

> Protein: 4 grams
> Carbohydrate: 41 grams

Fat: 12 grams

A bit of fat, but looks like a lot of carbos. Eat candy bars all day, and get healthy as a horse. A bit later he checked out a Hershey with Almonds.

Protein: 5 grams
Carbohydrates: 20 grams
Fat: 14 grams

Looks about the same so far. Then, under the carbohydrate category, the manufacturer listed a more detailed breakdown:

Sugar ....18 grams
Other Carbohydrates ......2 grams

How do you know whether a product you buy is listing simple or complex carbos on the labels? Try using your good judgement. If it is obvious that whatever you are buying is eighty percent sugar, and the label boasts of big numbers of carbos, use common sense. A candy bar is just that ... a candy bar

What's wrong with the "simple carbos," the ones that come sliding into home on the surface of a glazed doughnut, or a cream pie filling? Other than having next-to-zilch food value, sugars stimulate too much insulin. The insulin pulls too much glucose out of the blood and dumps it into the cells. Equating this to our engine/body comparison, it is like having the choke on all of the time in your engine. You get too rich a mixture with too much fuel in the carburetor. If you know anyone with diabetes, then you know how important the right fuel mixture in those microscopic cells can be.

Sugar isn't necessarily bad for you. Other than being a courier for a load of calories, it does not contain cholesterol or fat, so it won't cause heart disease, or cancer. It does not cause diabetes. It really doesn't do much for you, besides rotting your teeth, but you will find it almost impossible to avoid it. Most prepared food that you buy contains sugar in one form or another. For your own good, cut back on the really excessive sugar-dripping sweets. Compare it to a sexy member of the opposite sex overtly fondling your body at a cocktail party while your mate is in striking distance—nothing good can come of it, and for your own health, avoidance is highly advisable.

<u>Cholesterol</u>: This is the "killer," the "pipe-clogger," At least that is the impression given by some media hype and doomsayers. If your cholesterol level is over 200, you are suspect. If it is over 300 you should not feel safe unless you are within voice contact of a paramedic unit at all times. Just how "bad" is cholesterol? For the heck of it, let's create a worst-case scenario, using the previous "you" in the leading role. Your everyday diet is an absolute disaster, continually top-ending the fat ratio scale.

On this particular day, you really bend the needle:

Breakfast: Four eggs (fried), bacon, three doughnuts, coffee with two slugs of pure cream. Cholesterol count—about <u>1500mg</u> (milligrams)

Lunch: Two chicken liver sandwiches, heavy on the mayo, and a thick chocolate malt.
Cholesterol count—about <u>1200mg</u>

Dinner: You went totally crazy for dinner—deliciously prepared pork brains with all the trimmings. Well over <u>2000 mg</u> per serving, and, of course, you had seconds. Hold onto your hat. Cholesterol count—a whopping <u>4500mg</u>

Not good! Over 7000mg of cholesterol in a ten hour period. This doesn't even include all of the between-meal snacks that you invariably snuck in. Since the recommended daily intake of cholesterol is less than 300 mg you have knocked off enough for almost a whole month. With your blood pressure hovering at 210/95, your system is headed for overload … a complete meltdown, a la Chernobyl.

Later in the evening, while you are lounged out on the recliner, having just cracked open your third pack of unfiltered cigarettes, a beer in one hand, a handful of chocolate chip cookies in the other, watching a rerun of "Jake and the Fatman" it happens.

At first it feels like an elephant snuck into the room and sat on your chest. It is scary just visualizing it. Your hand clutches your chest, pain squirts up through your left shoulder and down into your arm. Your face contorts. Sweat pours off your body in buckets.

The next thing you know, people are poking needles in your arm, blowing in your mouth and beating on your chest. IV lines are sticking out of every major vein. The squiggles on the EKG scope are going up and down like a seismograph during a major earthquake. Then, zilch ... it's flat line.

You are history, man. You had the big one, the full-blown MI (Myocardial Infarction), coronary occlusion, etc. Hell, you didn't even rate a near-death experience. No bright lights, with the soft music and old friends at the end of the tunnel. You snuffed too fast. Did too much cholesterol do you in? Nothing could get through the clogged up fuel lines to get to the old fuel pump. With the combination of pure-slob life style, sky-high blood pressure, massive cholesterol intake, and excessive booze and cigarettes, there is an odds-on chance that the assumption is correct. According to most of the experts on earth, you did just about everything possible to precipitate a fatal heart attack.

On the other hand, some interesting information regarding cholesterol and longevity has surfaced. For example, an article some years back in Readers Digest disclosed fascinating insights. It appears that people with extremely low blood-cholesterol levels, precisely, those with below 160 were at low risk for heart disease, but may get nailed from another angle. The studies concluded that men with low cholesterol were up to three times as likely to suffer a hemorrhagic stroke—a ruptured blood vessel in the brain (nice thought), and twice as likely to be diagnosed with cancer.

Turn you life upside down trying to build a healthy heart, and then find out that you are liable to get blind-sided by a couple of other killers. Studies concluded that, "men with cholesterol in the 160 to 220 range had substantially fewer deaths from all causes than did men above or below those levels." So, guys, if your cholesterol level is above 220, you know what you have to do. Faithfully follow the tidbits of healthful habits that you have learned from this book.

If your level is below 160, well, you know what to do ... slam-dunk a half gallon of rocky road ice cream every day. Just kidding. You should consider the following

Milk: Some studies have linked fat with cancer, including cancer of the colon. Since whole milk (the rich, tasty kind) is the reportedly a big source of saturated fat in the so-called average diet, it would seem whole milk is definitely suspect in the colon cancer caper. On the other hand some research has reportedly shown that low-fat milk can be a cancer fighter.

1. Drinking whole milk may be a factor in causing cancer.

2. Drinking low-fat or non-fat milk may help avoid the same cancer.

3. Drinking no milk at all is riskier, cancer-wise, than drinking whole milk.

Conclusion? Try the 1% milk. It keeps looking better all the time.

Still not convinced that the benefits of healthy eating are worth exchanging for the pleasure you derive from that high-cholesterol, super-rich, fat-bloated mess you call a diet? You should think about the following. There is a good chance that the same occlusions that are clogging your larger arteries, are doing likewise to the smaller ones, such as ... the penis arteries. If you picked up on the hows and whys of hardons discussed earlier, then it shouldn't take a PHD to realize that ... no blood—no boner, even with Viagra or one of its cousins. The condition is called *arterial impotence*, caused by a narrowing of the internal pudendal artery and its branches. Guess what causes this unfortunate condition? How about an accumulation of FAT on the artery walls? This is an unfortunate fact of life for many of the limp-rods running loose today. The choice is yours!

AND SEX FOREVER

CHAPTER 12

SPECIAL EXERCISES FOR YOUR "SEX MUSCLES"

How many of you turned to this chapter first? Nothing to be ashamed of … you are probably not alone. It is highly likely that many people would have checked this section of the book first. Conversely, if you catch your teenage daughter and her friends studying this chapter, you may want to admonish them sternly. They should be ashamed of themselves. They could be doing something constructive—like watching MTV.

What and where are these so-called "sex muscles?" If we broaden the interpretation of what constitutes "sex," the answer becomes more complex. Some think of sex only in terms of humping and thumping. A slow, sensual, head-to-toe body massage could be closer to pure sex than a no-brainer mattress romp.

So, there is really no precise answer. It is true that some muscle groups are used strictly for getting the pile driver going, but there are others with action so subtle that no visible movement is involved. Guys, if you have been hoping that there are some secret exercises that will give you a schlong like an Italian salami, sorry, it just ain't gonna happen. You can try one of those Vac-U-Sucks advertised in the back pages of men's girly magazines. They may not work, but they do have their fringe benefits. Recently an M.D. on a TV infomercial was touting a device that looked suspiciously like one of those things, and he claimed that it works wonders for treating impotence. Hell, who knows?

Remember the old saying, God created all men equal? You might have believed that, until your first high school gym class hit the showers. Then you discovered that, in his infinite wisdom, he created some more equal than others. Well, there is really not much one can do in this respect, so instead, you make the most of what you have. Undoubtedly, you have heard another old chestnut ... "It ain't the meat, it's the motion," obviously originated by one of the lesser endowed. Actually, there is a whole lot of truth in this old chestnut. There are exercises that may increase your performance, your sexual vigor, your longevity (and her appreciation). And, yes, they are covered later in this book. But, before we get into these little gems, let's take a behind the scenes look at how the male sex machine works.

The supposedly highly complex sexual response system of the male of the human species is not really so complex. In fact, it is actually very simple. It can be broken down into two basic activities:

1. Getting Roger rigid, and
2. Getting the proper fluids moving

The primary stimulation necessary to start Roger rising to rigidity depends on a lot of things, such as age, physical condition, sexual preference, etc. A 17-year-old male has more of a problem keeping it down than he does in getting it up. A 75-year-old man may pray a lot.

Here is how it works. For illustration purposes, let us assume that you are a normal, red blooded, healthy guy. You spot some great T and A, and your imagination goes to work. This information goes directly to the horny part of the brain, the cortex. The cortex digests this data, and then sends a memo by messenger down the hall to the hypothalamus. Here the big decision is made ... are you worthy and deserving of a full-blown erection? Now, your hypothalamus has a lot of other, more important things to do—like regulate breathing, heart rate, body temperature, hunger, thirst, etc ... so you better have some darn good stimulation going to get its attention. For the ladies, the hypothalamus produces a hormone called oxytocin, known as the "hormone of love," which affects female lactation and those "sexy" feelings.

If you get the go-ahead, you lucky devil, the messenger heads south down the spinal cord, through the sacral nerves to the control panel that controls a sphincter muscle (not the sphincter muscle. That one is located at the tip of your exhaust pipe). This one encircles your penis artery and is usually clamped shut. Guess what happens when this sphincter muscle loosens up. Yea! A heavy load of oxygenated blood starts a code 3 response through your crotch, past that loosened sphincter, engorges the soft, spongy tissue found occupying the region, and Roger swells majestically. Remember Viagra and its relatives? Basically, all they do is open the flood gates and let the oxygenated blood flow. Then the little sphincter tightens up just enough to keep that wonderful blood trapped. Phase one is complete.

Now for Phase Two. About halfway between the testicles and the anal sphincter lies a gland about the size of a ping-pong ball. This is your prostate. Some young guys aren't too familiar with their prostate, but you can damn well believe that they will be as they get a little older. Some day, a doctor is going to say, "Bend over and grab you ankles." Hang on tight, Brother. You are about to experience the finger-wave. He is getting ready to check your prostate for unusual lumps or enlargement. Without surgery there is only one way to get there. You guessed it. God, what an uncomfortable feeling. Most doctors have fingers the size of thumbs.

This little gland is the center of attention in the three-ring circus of sexual stimulation. It has a lot of duties. It monitors activities in the southern sector, in direct communication with the cortex. It is always on alert, ready to spring into action. All it needs is the right signal from the brain. When the hypothalamus makes the decision to go for it, the prostate is notified immediately. A batch of fluid is put in the mixer and the testicles snap to attention, ready for mobilization.

By now, Roger is fully rigid. On the underside of the tip of Rogers knob is a highly sensitive nerve center. After sufficient titillation on this nerve center, the prostate goes into action. The muscles around the gland start to squeeze rhythmically. The prostrate squishes like an orange and the fluid starts to move, picks up speed, sucking millions of squirming little spermatozoa into the stream with, basically, a venturi effect (remember Physics I in high school). This volatile mixture flows though the rigid digit until it explodes into orgasmic freedom.

So, you are thinking. B.F.D. Who cares? As long as the equipment works who gives a rat's ass how it does it? Well Amigo, you should! The sexual response system is an important ally—treat it right, and it will serve you will until you die of old age. Abuse it, and you could be sorry. There are a lot of miserable souls, and I don't mean just old farts, who find to their dismay that the only time Roger comes to life is around 3 a.m. when the bladder is full. This condition results in the proverbial "piss hardon". No erotic stimulation involved—you could be dreaming about changing oil in your car. The response system is relaxed while you are asleep and sometimes may get fooled by pressure from the bladder.

There you sit, proud as hell, with this "woody." Wanting to share the event with your loved one, you give her a gentle nudge and say, "Hey, Babe, take a look at this beauty." At that time of morning, her probable response would be something like "You disgusting pig." Undaunted, you reach over for a little feely. For most guys, foreplay isn't a big consideration at 3 a.m. If you don't get smacked, you will at least be greeted with "get your goddam hands off me, you friggin' pervert."

Do you suffer from an uncooperative, unresponsive, unwilling weenie? Intermittent impotence. The big "I." Summed up graphically many years ago by an infamous West Coast philosopher and radio DJ, Robert W. Morgan (that the author, years ago, listened to while driving to UCLA) with the following axiom of wisdom:

> Question—What is the difference between anxiety and panic?
> Answer—*Anxiety* is the first time you can't do it the second time.
> *Panic* is the second time you can't do it the first time.

Don't let this happen to you. There is no reason it should happen to you. What can one do, you ask? There is no simple, single answer. There are several things you can do. The sex exercises you will be doing can help. What you eat is important. Your blood pressure is important. Whether or not you smoke is important. Drugs and booze can play a negative roll. So, get ready to activate your sexual prowess to its maximum capability.

Bumps and Grinds

Some of the exercises utilized to stimulate and activate the muscle groups referred to here as the "sex muscles" are patterned after the basic down and dirty vaudevillian strippers' bump and grind routine. If you have never had the opportunity to view a good stripper in action, then you have missed out on a memorable experience. The author's introduction to this fascinating world occurred while he was still in high school. Four or five of "the boys" piled into the car and headed for the Follies Burlesque, 5th and Main, downtown L.A. skid row. They grabbed seats in the front row with all of the bald-headed guys and hooted and hollered like a bunch of fools.

The headliner that night was Tempest Storm, a statuesque, flaming red head, built like a brick you-know-what. She was beautiful. What a body—a true study in anatomic perfection.

And what breasts. It would have been a dishonor to call those beauties pectorals. They were not merely breasts, either—gorgeous, ripe melons, all natural, one hundred percent Grade A, FDA approved, organically grown, no plastic added. The kind men would like to have a half-acre of to run across barefooted, and crawl back on their hands and knees. To top it off, her breasts were trained. She could make her tassels swing in a circle together in the same direction, then in the opposite direction, and even stop one or the other at will. She moved as gracefully as a cat. She didn't just follow the music—she was welded to it. Every movement was in perfect sync to the distinctive drumbeat.

The thought of actually having sexual contact with this goddess of female beauty was beyond the scope of ones limited imagination. It was once reported by informed sources that she had her body insured for a million dollars. Tempest Storm gave an unforgettable demonstration of the proper use of bumps and grinds. So, exactly what are the bumps and grinds?

> Bumping is simply using the pelvic muscles to thrust the hip and groin portion of the anatomy forward and backward.

> Grinding is using the same muscles to rotate the same portions of the anatomy in a circular motion-round and round.

For the guys It is pretty basic and reverts to the old axiom—"it ain't the meat, it's the motion." This means that size alone is not the most important criteria. If you take a few straight in-and-out pokes, finish, then roll over to watch more TV, or start snoring, don't be surprised if your lady seems to have a lot of door-to-door salesman stopping by while you're at work. You just need to do some of the exercises in this chapter to have her screaming with delight.

For the Gals We are going to venture into an age-old fantasy that men throughout the world might discuss amongst themselves. Discussing this could be a little sensitive. The simplest explanation is the ability of a woman to control and regulate "rhythmic muscular contractions." Disgusting, gross? Not really. Sexual muscular control can be achieved. Some of the exercises about to be described might help to achieve this revered status.

Basic B and G

Unless you happen to be a natural extrovert with a flair for the bizarre, especially guys, you will feel like a foolish jerk when you practice the basic bump and grind movements. Standing in the middle of a room humping the air is an unusual activity in anyone's book. If it helps, you can close your eyes and fantasize that you are the hottest ticket at a sexy night club, turning on a room full of sweaty, screaming, horny women.

Gals, taking a shot at emulating Gypsy Rose Lee (She was once the Goddess of Strippers, who was immortalized by Natalie Wood in the movie "Gypsy") should give you a bit of a vicarious thrill. So, <u>put on some sinful music</u>, unwind and let yourself go! Or, you can tune in to MTV and try to keep up with the stimulating motions of the younger set.

The Basic Bump is just that, the old fashioned burlesque "bump." To begin, you stand in one place with your legs spread a few inches, knees bent slightly, and you move your pelvic region forward and backward. Occasionally, as you near the finish of the forward movement, give a vigorous thrust with the groin. After you get into this exercise with vigor and enthusiasm, you will find that you can get some interesting hand and arm motion into the action. For example, clasping your hands behind the back of neck while you pump back and forth, or placing one or both hands on the cheeks of your fanny can feel downright nasty.

There are four different variables: long, short, fast and slow. Try each in different combinations. For example, begin with long, slow movements—move your derriere to the rear, arching your back at the same time. Then, reverse the action with a hard forward thrust.

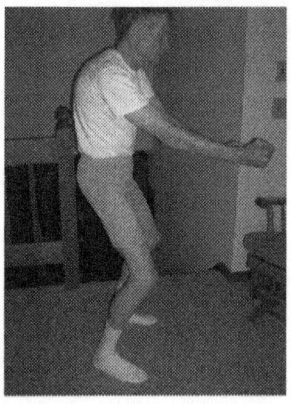 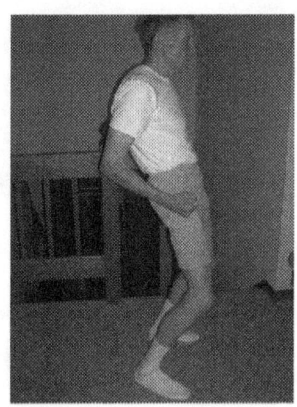

Back and forth, back and forth.
Try it fifteen or twenty times.

Now, some short, quick strokes. Turn up the volume on the music. Pop
that pelvic portion fore and aft with gusto. Powerful, vicious thrusts.
Grunt a little. Grit your teeth.
Hump! Hump! Hump!

See how long you can keep it going before your muscles start to cramp. Try it for
two full minutes on the clock. You have been bragging all these years about how
you can do it for hours. Maybe it just seemed like hours.

The other two combinations are:
  1. Long, fast strokes and
  2. Short, slow strokes

Mix and match. Try all of the combinations. It shouldn't be too long before you realize how this entertaining activity can be put to good use in other areas of your life.

The Basic Grind You assume the same initial position as for the Bump. Same
variables—long, short, fast and slow. The only difference is the movement. But,
viva la difference. The grind can be a sexual experience in itself. To begin, move
the hips to the left as far as possible, then in a circular movement forward and all
the way to the right. Then move the hips to the rear as far as possible as you continue the circular action.

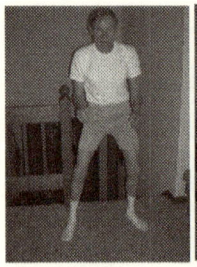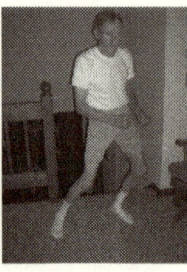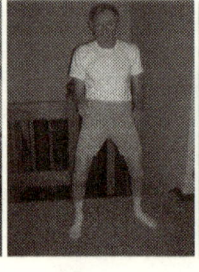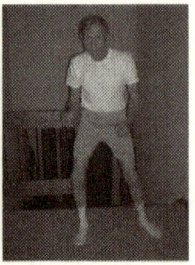

A peculiar phenomena surfaces when men are rotating their mid-sections in
grind-like movements while they are dancing. Some of them circulate their fannies clockwise, some counter-clockwise. Maybe it has something to do with left-
hang, right-hang. Or how about which way you rotated while sliding headfirst

down the birth canal? Who knows! This could be a great topic for an in-depth, federally funded research study.

Just for the hell of it, find out which way you swing (sorry, poor choice of words). Go ahead. Crank your pelvis in a circular movement. Which direction did it head? More than likely it will travel in the same orbit every time you put it in motion. Even so, it is more effective to give it a try in both directions when doing the **basic grind**.

Start off with a slow, short circle. Go up on your toes as you rotate to the front. This gives your calves a little work, and makes the act look more wanton and lustful. Keep it up for about a minute. Then switch directions. Feel gawky? That's OK. Go at it for another minute or so. Now, open it up. Keep it slow, but make it a big, wide arc. All the way around—up on the toes—try giving the pelvis a healthy forward thrust as you near the frontal lobe of the big swing. Put in some sound effect with the hearty thrust—like the swish of a drummer rapping his cymbal with a brush. Change directions again, and keep up the swishing.

Step on the throttle—smaller rotations, but turn up the heat. Don't stop the swish—it should sound like a machine gun as you pick up steam. Suck the gut in as you go around. Slow down long enough to change directions and then rev through the gears.

Finally, you can start easing into a longer arc with gusto. Fast, big circles—up on the toes. Switch directions a little sooner with this routine.

Well that's it. As you get more proficient with the Basic Bump and Grind you will find yourself experimenting with combinations of all the movements ... change the tempo, the action, more sound effects, soft thrusts, hard thrusts, erotic and exotic arm and body movements. Go for it. You may find some pleasing rewards for your effort.

The Erotic Door Knob

If you think you looked weird humping thin air with the basic bump and grind, wait until you try the doorknob routines. You definitely do not want to be surprised by anyone while you are into this action (especially someone who has any reservations regarding you sanity and/or your stability). The necessary apparatus is one standard interior-type door with doorknobs on both sides of the door. The only other criterion is that the doorknobs be sturdy and pretty close to crotch-height.

Open the door far enough to give yourself ample room to maneuver. Stand facing the edge of the door, your hands grasping both sides of the doorknob. Next, plant your feet on both sides of the door about a foot or so apart. Now comes the weird part. Bend your knees, and lean back until your arms are straight. From this very abnormal position, you can bump and grind to your hearts content. Again privacy is a must. An unwitting observer might think that you have really lost it this time.

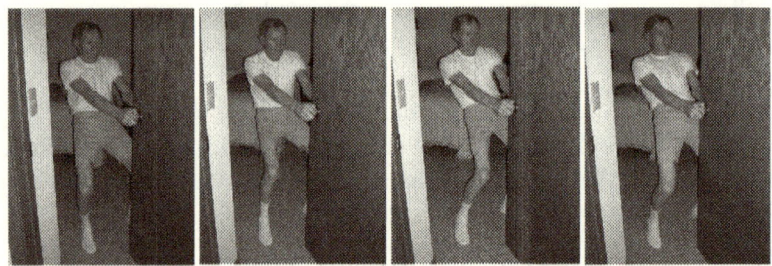

You can perform all bump and grind movements: fast, slow, long and short. You can vary the routine by changing the amount of knee-bend and thus the angle of your body. If you feel really athletic, you can lean way back until your body is almost parallel with the ground.

Have some fun while you are into these maneuvers. Let go with one hand, and place the other somewhere else—such as the back of your neck, the back of your head, or, if you happen to feel exceptionally uninhibited, on the back of your buns.

You can simulate sensory gratification by the way you hold the doorknob. If you grab it with your palms down, you aren't using much imagination.

Try grabbing it from the ends, with your palms facing each other. Doesn't that feel a little more perverse? Your stimulus can really increase if you grasp it palms-up, with a slight bend at the elbows.

If you don't feel like you are performing an enticing, sensuous act, you need to double-check your vitamin intake.

How long you can do the erotic doorknob bump and grind routine depends on how much knee-bend you use, how far you lean back, and how vigorously you pursue the movements. Thirty seconds to a minute should be more than ample. Remember to suck in the gut and tighten the buns. Your pelvic muscles, thighs, lower back, glutes and even your biceps and shoulders will benefit from all of this sensuous action.

The Jack Hammer

Not everyone will find this exercise to his or her liking. Especially if one has great globs of girth surrounding the middle of the body. In fact, it could be downright dangerous to the participant and anyone else within the structure inhabited by the participant. The object of the Jack Hammer is to tense up your pelvic area so completely that this portion of the body begins to quiver and shake with a tremulous motion. Getting the action going is a little like starting the engine in your car. You keep cranking it until it catches hold and takes off by itself. You may even get your whole body involved

The best position for doing the **Jack Hammer** is, for the lack of a formal name, the Incredible Hulk stance. If you are old enough to have watched that big green stud in action on your TV you will identify with the stance immediately. Legs spread, slight bend in the knees, eyes squinted, teeth clenched, arms out to the sides, every muscle in the body tensed. Next concentrate on getting the groin to quiver and shake until the pelvis is bouncing faster and faster. You might consider wearing a jock strap, or tight fitting underwear and shorts.

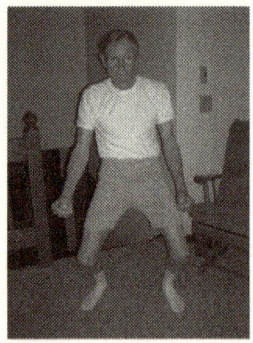

Don't feel rejected if you can't get the motion going at first. This is a rather peculiar movement, and again, privacy is recommended. If someone had doubts regarding your mental balance after observing you doing the erotic doorknob routine, a little peek at your **Jack Hammer** action would remove any remaining doubts.

It should be obvious in a hurry that a large jelly-belly could go seriously out of control during the **Jack Hammer** ... something like the marching troops breaking step when they cross a bridge so as to prevent a syncopated rhythm that could destroy the bridge. If you can keep the "Hammer" going for more than ten seconds, you are to be commended (and highly recommended). One can only imagine what would happen if a couple were coupled with both pelvises quivering away in a frantic **Jack Hammer** action.

You Do WHAT in Church?

You can do it while standing in line at the Post Office, at the bank, or the supermarket. You can even do it during hymns at church. People on either side of you won't know that you are doing it. If you are careful, and do it right, even those behind you can't tell. With a facade of nonchalance, you can look around, smile at people, and sing out with reverence and reverberation.

The Fifty-Cent Bun Squeezing Drill What you are doing can be referred to simply as **The Drill**. Many of these sex muscle routines are basically Kegel type exercise with some modifications. While standing, you tighten your cheeks (glutes). If you don't have a fifty-cent piece, pretend that you have one between them. Put a real good squeeze on. Hold it for as long as comfortable, and then gently relax. That's all there is to it. You can vary the procedure by alternately squeezing and relaxing, squeezing and relaxing, but when you do this you run the risk of exposure. Observant spectators to your rear can spot the crease of your pants repeatedly being sucked in, then releasing. If they are sharp, they will be thinking to themselves, "That guy in the aisle seat, row 5, is doing **The Drill**"

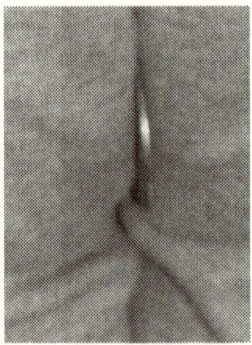

All the time a man is doing it, he is tightening and toughening some of the muscles that encompass that wonderful gland of gladness, the prostate. By now, you are certainly aware of the importance of a happy, healthy prostate. Notice that, in the process, a lot of other muscles get involved—the stomach (lower abdominals), the glutes (cheeks), the thighs, and some accessory muscles in the crotch area. Using the same process, the ladies can gain muscle control and stamina.

The Drill can be performed in the privacy of your usual workout location, actually using a fifty-cent piece. For the really adventurous, it could even be done in your birthday suit. Grab a coin and give it a try. If you are good, you can hold a quarter, a dime if you're really good.

Of course, while you are in church, or the supermarket, or the post office, you don't actually place a coin between your cheeks, nor do you drop your drawers. You just imagine that a coin is there, and squeeze accordingly.

Do it with Music

If you want to see something strange, try watching those TV dance/exercise gurus with the sound muted. Their jerking and bouncing looks really strange without musical accompaniment. It is true, though, that music helps. In fact, it can really get your motor revved up. Oldies rock and roll is the greatest. Crank up the volume on a chorus of *Old Time Rock and Roll,* and if you don't leap up and bump, hump and grind all over the room you are a born zero. Millions of women almost went into heat when they watched the movie *Risky Business* with Tom Cruise gliding across the floor in his underwear, shaking his hips suggestively to—you guessed it—Bob Seger's *Old Time Rock and Roll.* Or, how about Patrick Swayze *Dirty Dancing* up a storm with Cynthia Rhodes and Jennifer Grey? Richard Gere and Jennifer Lopez worked up quite a sweat in *Shall We Dance.* TVs *Dancing With the Stars* has had some real talent. Great moves by all.

Try any of the sex muscle movements to the down-and-dirty beat of *Night Train* and feel the action. Go on—accentuate those bumps and grinds. Fantasize a little. It's free, and you never know what your imagination can come up with. What's that you say? Your belly keeps moving west after your hips are headed back to the east. So, who cares? You're having fun and it's good for you. This is a hard confession to make, but occasionally I find myself watching MTV. (That's American Bandstand with an "X" rating.) You see some sexually explicit stuff, with great hip movement. Most interesting though are the gymnastic gyrations associated with the newer art forms—rap and hip-hop. You have to be one hell of an athlete to keep up with the good rap and hip-hop dancers. Who knows, a movement may be started to have them included as an event in the next Olympics.

Chapter 13

It's Party Time

Who says you can't have fun while you are getting fit? You can party down, chase skirts (or pants), shake your bootie, and get healthy in the process. To do so involves some discipline and moderation. It also stands to reason that if you free-base coke all day and shoot heroin all night, you are not displaying discipline and moderation.

On the other hand, you aren't training for the Olympics either. You are doing all of this routine so you can feel better, look better, live longer, love longer and enjoy life to the max. If it means that you have to become a tee totaling, celibate wallflower, then maybe fitness for you is not so wonderful after all. Is there a happy medium? How much is too much, how much is too little? Let's look at the variables.

Demon Rum

Can a little booze actually be good for you? It doesn't seem likely since, every year, thousands of otherwise decent citizens pickle their livers, or get juiced and kill off their fellow humans at an astonishing rate while trying to control a two-ton 4-wheeled guided missile. Others just sit around getting sloshed, and screw up their own lives and the lives of everyone around them.

If you discount those poor souls who have a problem handling the stuff in any quantity, then you may be surprised to learn that two drinks a day may be better for you than no drinks at all. Some studies concluded that two ounces of alcohol, taken over an extended period of time in a day aided in relaxation, stress reduction and, get this, a decrease in heart disease. Note that it said "over an extended period of time." Two ounces of undiluted hard liquor, downed in one gulp on an empty stomach, may knock you right straight on your ass. I will guarantee that it won't do your heart any good.

Results of the study produced an interesting curve. It would appear that those who shun the fluid completely tend to be more uptight, and their fuel pump breaks down more often than the two-ounce drinkers. Statistically, there was not too much difference, but the two-ounce a day crowd did show less tendency to heart disease than the total abstainers.

Now, going the other way, the curve really takes off in the wrong direction. Take three or more ounces a day continuously and your body can get trashed in a big hurry.

Is this an endorsement for the use of alcohol as an adjunct to becoming physically fit?

No way. If you don't imbibe now, don't show classic stupidity and start to drink just because some weirdo doctor claims that two ounces of hooch a day is beneficial. Get serious. Most mature adults (and many immature ones) have an occasional drink. But, too many already drink too much. How much is too much? Well, apparently anything more than two ounces a day is too much. More than that may damage the body, and, guys, it can adversely affect you in a very personal way. Most men who have, at one time or another, indulged much too heavily, have discovered that an interesting but rather embarrassing condition can arise. In their minds, they feel like a raging stud bull. But down south a different message is being received To begin with, alcohol can act as a stimulant as well as a depressant (a biphasic response)—it gets the heart jumping and the blood flowing. So, if the blood is pumping at a rapid pace the hypothalamus (remember him?) has its hands full, and the vital message to the tightened sphincter above the crotch may not get sent. The blood goes everywhere but "there."

Have you ever experienced the futility of trying to talk that thing up? Good luck! Worse yet, how about closing the eyes and trying to think it up? Absolute futility! Even if a little blood slipped through and Roger started to rise, the alcohol in the system could unexpectedly and suddenly shift gears and start reacting as a depressant. Even if one were lucky enough to get it up, one might be too relaxed to use it.

In reality, you really are not having fun if you are blotto drunk. Instead:

> You stink,
> You make an ass out of yourself, and
> You wake up the next morning with a swollen head, a belly full of puke, and the feeling that a flock of pigeons took a dump in your mouth.

Remember discipline and moderation? After finishing two drinks, switch to soda water with a twist of lime. Then you can sit back and watch the pigeons circle over someone else's mouth.

The Benefits of Smoking

Everyone is always ragging on smoking. Restaurants, public buildings, and airlines all are against smokers. Doctors make derogatory claims about smoking being unhealthy, obnoxious and dangerous. If anything, we here in the U.S. don't smoke enough—the average smoker in Russia supposedly spends as much as 10% of his income on the weed. So, get with it. Light up. We can't let those Ruskies beat us in anything.

Actually, when you think about it, there are a lot of benefits to smoking:

> 1. Smoking provides a true test for your home smoke detector. Pushing that little red button ever so often does not prove anything, except that the buzzer makes noise. An occasional cigarette left in a couch, an overstuffed chair or your pillow provides a more positive test ... real fire, along with real smoke.

> 2. Old people are a burden on society. They shuffle around aimlessly, snot running out of their nose, complaining, messing their pants all of the time. If you are twenty years old and smoke, you won't have to worry about such indignities. Actuarially, you should be pushing up daisies somewhere around the age of 64. You might consider appealing to Social Security for an exemption from their ridiculously high SSA payroll tax? You won't need the benefits anyway. You can be a true patriot, turning down all of those government handouts. Now, look at that non-smoking high and mighty neighbor of yours. He should be slopping at the federal money trough until he is at least 83, keeping his heirs waiting forever for their rightful inheritance.

3. Smokers are much more likely to continue weightlifting in their waning years. A high percentage of them wind up connected to a large green steel tank of pure oxygen. These tanks are not light. A good, sturdy 66 cubic foot capacity bottle can weigh well over 100 pounds. Dragging that sucker around everywhere you go is no easy task. Oddly enough, most smokers who find themselves in this condition (a little emphysema here, a little lung cancer there) have only one pleasure in life ... that being their next smoke. But, if you think about it for a minute, what else do they have to look forward to? Sex is history, they can't travel, and tennis and golf are out. They do have to be careful around the O-2 though ... lighting up in an oxygen enriched atmosphere could send the tank shooting into the night sky like a scud missile with the smoker still attached by his plastic tube.

4. Smoking works wonders for ones appearance. Notice the distinctive characteristics that distinguish the smoker. A sexy, light yellow tint on the teeth; deep, sensuous wrinkles on the graying facial skin; white ashes flicked all over their brand new navy-blue outfit, resembling a personal snowstorm.

5. That dry, hacking cough with a gross ball of smoky phlegm can get one out of lots of situations, such as: speaking engagements, dinner with a gorgeous blind date, asking for a raise, etc.

6. You never find yourself in that embarrassing situation where you don't know what to do with your hands. And, at the same time you satisfy the craving your mouth has developed—having something in it all the time. The poor non-smoker is at a loss. You can't sit there and play with yourself. And a guy looks a little weird if he sits daintily with his hands folded neatly on his lap.

7. You can be cool. Check out those studs in the magazine and TV ads—shirt open, hairy, muscular chest, strong, jutting dimpled chin (a la Kirk Douglas), care-free to-hell-with-the-world attitude. All of that can be yours (if you buy the right brand, naturally). Young girls, you should pay attention. Nothing in the world looks quite like a woman taking a big drag on a cigarette. Guys really dig on kissing a girl who just finished one—about as much as licking an ash tray.

The satire above is not going to cause anyone to turn over a new leaf and give up the nicotine, one of the strongest addictive substance known. If you are a smoker, even if you won't admit it, you know that it is screwing up your health big time. You either don't give a damn, or can't and won't do anything about it. But you really don't have to worry about your particular breed of addiction going away too soon. Each day, more than three thousand teens and younger children reportedly start sucking the weed. Gets them a good head start on blackened, leathery lungs.

I did try to come up with something positive about smoking. Unfortunately, there is nothing positive to be found. In fact, the more research the more the bad news surfaced, such as the fact that smokers have a much greater chance of getting cancer.

If you don't like your family, by all means be sure you continue smoking. Lots of evidence shows that secondary smoke (the nasty stuff that you exhale) is pretty much as bad for everyone around you as the stuff that you inhaled is for you. Even your little sprouts can share the benefits. Merry Christmas, kids—Daddy is giving all of us a nice respiratory infection this year.

Rock Around the Clock

Remember the old joke about the very woeful, very pregnant young maiden who sang "I Should Have Danced All Night?" Well, so should you. As we discussed earlier dancing is a great aerobic-type exercise. Look at Fred Astaire. He didn't have an ounce of fat on him. He was one lean, mean, dancing machine. Guys, if you want to score some real points with your loved one, take her out to dance. Almost all women love to dance. She will love you for it.

> You don't dance? Learn. Take it up A.S.A.P.
> You're too old to learn how to dance? B.S.!

> Look around at some of the old geezers that are as spry as chickens, and you can bet they still get out and hoof it whenever they get the chance. If she doesn't know how to dance, have her take some lessons with you. It's more fun that way, anyhow. The dividends will greatly outweigh the investment.

> By dancing, we mean <u>dancing</u>. Moving vigorously around the floor— working up a sweat. If you are one of those Rudolph Vaselino types that stand in one place, move slightly to every fourth or fifth beat of the music, eyes closed, your tongue buried an inch and a half into her ear,

glued crotch to crotch, both of your hands busy caressing and cupping the bottom of her buns ... you are not really dancing.

You are into a form of foreplay.

Now that is not all bad, and it definitely has its place in the whole scheme of things, but if it is the only ritual you can perform on the dance floor, you need to revise your game plan. Convinced? Good. What dances should you learn?

All of them. Foxtrot, cha-cha, rhumba, samba, tango, swing, rock and roll, any and all. You should also learn the two-step. Shit-kickers have one hell of a good time dancing, almost as much as they do drinking and fighting. If you do go to a country western bar, and you happen to think that some of the redneck patrons look a bit silly in their ten-gallon hats and their pointy-toed boots, discretion warrants keeping your thoughts to yourself. Especially if you are wearing horned-rim glasses, a gray three-piece business suit, and drinking a sloe gin fizz.

What is the best dance to get your main frame moving? How about the Twist. If you want to really cut loose, get down, and shake it around, do it to the Twist. You can almost feel the waistline shrinking while globules of fat ride piggyback on every sweat molecule flowing profusely out of your pores. If you were to do nothing else exercise-wise but Twist for twenty minutes every day, you couldn't help but knock off layers of unwanted blubber.

There is one thing about the Twist that seems a bit odd—Chubby Checker, the guy who started it all. Although he has trimmed up some since he first spilled onto the dance floors of America, by all rights, he should be Skinny Checker, the walking beanpole. Maybe he just had one hell of a ravenous appetite.

Other good dances? How about the Limbo Rock? Sensual, with a lot of good hip movement. Speaking of the Limbo Rock, a past experience exemplifies the benefits of dancing. On a week-end cruise from L.A. to Ensenada, it was Saturday night—the dress was formal, tuxes, evening gowns ... the whole nine yards. The dinner was great. For desert, the chef turned out Baked Alaskan. For the less-than-sophisticates, that's a fancy ice cream cake with brandy poured on it. Then it is torched and the brandy burns off. Very impressive. Before serving it, all of the waiters formed a line, each carrying a cake, and then they marched through the aisles, moving to the Limbo Rock. The last waiter in line was a Jamaican fellow with shoulders a block wide, a 25 inch waist, and *really* muscular glutes (butt muscles) that were covered with skin-tight black satin pants that looked like they had been painted on.

This guy had at least six forward and two reverse speeds in his gear box. His hip action resembled two wildcats fighting in a gunnysack—a fact that did not go unnoticed by the hundred or so ladies dining at the time. There was no mistaking where he was in the room. All you had to do was follow the chorus of gasps, shrieks, and squeals. He didn't speak much English, but his body language was universal. It was quite a sight, watching dignified women reaching out and trying to feel his buns, or actually getting up and suggestively wiggling their fannies behind him—in their full dress formal attire.

See what you are missing out on. Dancing is fun, it's cheap, highly appreciated by your partner, and great for the slow-twitch muscle fibers.

In Bed—With His Boots On

Ask any man, if he had a choice, how he would prefer to leave this earth, and his likely response would be—ninety years old, in the sack with a 21 year old Playboy Centerfold, getting it on for Old Glory. Which brings up the question, how dangerous is the down-and-dirty, mattress-squashing, breath-gasping, really sweaty act of vigorous sexual intercourse?

It is great fun. It makes you feel good. And, in reality, it is pretty much what this whole mess is all about, is it not? But, is it good for you? Does it help-or—hinder a fitness program? Would you live longer if you were neutered just prior to puberty? Whether or not sex affects athletic performance has been debated for a long time. Actually, the debate is backwards ... we should be more concerned about whether or not athletic performance affects sex.

In the 1950's there was a serious young body-builder—advocate of vitamins, wheat germ, brewers yeast (yuk), the whole shot—who claimed that sex was seriously detrimental to male athletic performance. At the time some folklore had it that losing a CC (cubic centimeter) of jizz (the code name then for male ejaculate) was the equivalent of losing a pint of blood. Many a young athlete was terrified. Some had not even experienced sex yet and then to find out that dreaming about it could be physically debilitating was a truly crushing blow. Every night before a big sports event many would pray ... "Please Lord, no wet dreams tonight, I can't afford to give up eight pints of blood." Incidentally, did you know that some boxers, to this day, supposedly pack ice around their balls the night before a fight to ward off unwanted nocturnal emissions? Can you believe that?

Maybe they plan to cold-cock their opponent.
So, what is the true scoop?
Does it or doesn't it?

Believe it or not, after all these years, the jury is still out, but it is leaning towards acquittal. The American Medical Association, a few years back, concluded that sex the night before competition is not harmful, unless:

      1.) The athlete does not get enough sleep;
      2.) Is not used to having sex; or
      3.) Honestly believes that sex will impair his or her performance.

Then again who really cares about what does or does not affect world class athletes? How about the run-of-the-mill, out-of-shape ordinary everyday guys and gals? Is the old in-and-out going to hasten us to an early grave?

Not necessarily—unless one happens to be a total misfit trying to keep up with a twenty-one year old nymphomaniac. And even in this situation, the Creator had the foresight to install a shut-off valve somewhere in the limbic system. When you have had enough, Roger gets benched. Even so, if you try hard enough, you can still screw yourself to death. It will just take longer.

Sex itself is not at all harmful to the health. Casey Stengel, legendary manager of the New York Yankees, put things in proper perspective when, referring to his ballplayers, he replied, in so many words, "It ain't sex that wrecks these guys, it's chasing around all night looking for it."

How about females? It is no contest, fellows. The ladies can outlast us every time. Except for an occasional tune-up and lube job, the female apparatus pretty much has a lifetime, factory warranty. You may abuse it, but you will have a tough time breaking it. So ... a quiet evening, a cocktail or two by candlelight, slow dancing to soft music, a little neck-kissing and ear nibbling, a caress here and there, instant evaporation of unnecessary garments ... then, statistically, five to seven minutes in the standard missionary position, burning up approximately 200 to 300 calories, is not going to do you harm.

On the other hand, guys—chasing around to every meat-market singles bar in town, hound-dogging anything and everything that wears a skirt, powering down shooters and slammers with both hands, all in a smoke-filled atmosphere totally devoid of oxygen (and striking out continuously using every canned line in the book)—that's harmful and stressful. And what if you do happen to score?

After eight to ten hours of such destructive behavior, you might need two popsicle sticks and a roll of scotch tape to do anyone any good ... including yourself.

CHAPTER 14

THE ONLY SAFE SEX IS PHONE SEX

When the author was about four years old his father moved the family to the State of Washington. While living there they used the STD... meaning *Seattle Transit District* to get where they were going. Of course, today STD means Sexually Transmitted Diseases—absolutely no connection to Seattle's excellent bus system.

Safe sex is the "in" thing. This is not really a new concept. The author's generation was concerned about safe sex, but it had a different meaning then—like not getting caught by her old man (father, husband or boy friend, whichever the case). Now, you may be thinking, "What does all of this have to do with fitness?"

Hopefully, nothing. But, if you are unattached, or married and carousing on the sly, you better pay close attention and be careful where you go poking around. With your newly found virility comes a large amount of responsibility. In essence you are equipped with a lethal weapon and probably should be required to have a license of some sort before being allowed to use it. First is the obvious possibility of impregnating some unsuspecting female. Second, and equally important, is the prolific spread of sexually transmitted diseases because they actually can be lethal.

Hong Cong Dong

STDs have been around for a long time. Maybe you saw movies about them in high school health class or the military. Today, kids may spend a quarter of P.E. classes learning about STDs. The best special effects people in Hollywood couldn't possibly duplicate the horror and gore of bodies covered with puss-filled sores, mutilated flesh and gangrenous genitals. Seeing those flicks should have been enough to guarantee lifetime celibacy. But, alas, penis erectus has no conscience, so we may have worried about picking up a dose, but, unfortunately, most guys did not worry about it until after the fact. For example, take the fable about the businessman who traveled to an Asian country and decided to try a little strange stuff. After he returned home he discovered that his wand was turning purple and his foreskin was peeling off. His doctor told him that he had picked up a rare Asian venereal disease called Hong Kong Dong. It was incurable and they would have to amputate. He tried two other doctors—same diagnosis—amputation. In desperation he looked up an old Chinese healer. "Yes, it Hong Kong Dong," the healer said. "But American doctor knife happy, always cut, cut, cut… No need amputate. Wait two week … it fall off by self."

So, you see, no one is immune from the threat. When the author was a young buck, unencumbered and full of piss and vinegar, he met a sexy looking thing in a bowling alley bar called, get this, the *Beaver Room*. After two beers and some smooth talk (isn't it funny that, no matter how pickled one may get, they will swear that they only had two beers?) they wound up at her place. After a few kisses articles of clothing started coming off. To make a long story short, when she removed one of her shoes the top of her foot sported the grossest sore imaginable. She said that she cut herself shaving her legs.

Yeah, sure, lady! The author made up some phony excuse and made a hasty exit. Never mind its unusual location—by the time he got in to see a doctor his imagination had this slime-laden sore built up to be the King Kong of VD. All he had done was kiss her, but he was positive that millions of germs had osmosed through the mucous membranes of his mouth, and within days his brain would be ravaged with lesions.

The doctor was quite amused. The author wasn't. Doc asked only one question, "Where did you kiss her?" On the mouth, stupid. He said not to worry, but strongly advised avoiding the Beaver Room. The author wasn't convinced, and continued to study the surface of his body intensely, watching for tell-tale weird sores. He was in a state of panic for six months.

Whatever you call it, it is really no laughing matter. They have diseases now that are not even pronounceable, let alone curable. And, seriously, today, with sexual activity beginning at much earlier ages, sexually transmitted diseases are as big of a problem as ever. The responsibility lies with both partners, but guys, you can't afford not to afford condoms (We'll discuss that later). So, let's take a look at what's really out there:

AIDS In the fall of 1991 professional basketball star Ervin "Magic" Johnson boldly stepped forward and set the world on its ear by disclosing that he was HIV positive... he had contracted AIDS. It can be said that with this courageous act by one of the most popular athletes of all time brought this terrible STD out of the closet. It was no longer a forgotten problem in far off sub-Saharan Africa, a "gay scourge" or a needle-head drug addict's stupidity. Anyone could be infected. Just what are AIDS and HIV anyway? Acquired Immune Deficiency Syndrome (AIDS) is the result of symptoms and infections from the damage to a person's immune system from invasion of HIV, the human immunodeficiency virus, which is the other collection of letters from the alphabet soup. It can invade you from almost any available orifice or any bodily fluid, including mother to baby during pregnancy. Existing treatments can slow down the progress of the virus, but there is no known cure as yet. It is becoming an international crisis.

Gonorrhea It is sometimes known as the "clap." Guys may, for good reason, refer to it as the "drip." If you have it you will definitely know it. In about a week you experience what is incorrectly referred to as painful urination. It can go far beyond painful. If you have seen unusual very deep, long ridges forcefully scratched into the plaster above or beside a urinal or toilet—these could be tell-tale marks left by a clap-suffering male trying to take a simple pee. What finally is excreted might come out as greenish-yellow puss-like mucous. It is time to see a doctor, friend. Ditto for anyone you might have serviced in the previous six or seven days. Even though they may be spared the horrible pain at the potty, they are likely to get the worst of this one. A little discomfort, unusual discharge—maybe a little itch or redness. Not really uncommon problems for many gals. But, the after-affects are not nice. This germ can spread all over the place inside their body and wreak havoc... like being a very common cause of sterility. She might have to kiss motherhood bye-bye. Not a very sensible way to accomplish birth control. It can also cause PID (pelvic inflammatory disease) again with possible infertility, or, worst case scenario, ectopic pregnancy, a life-threatening condition. There is a closely related bug, now one of the most common crotch afflictions in the country, estimated three million new participants yearly, a real bad actor, sometimes mistaken for the clap… chlamydial infections.

Chlamydia This beauty is caused by principally the same germ that causes conjunctivitis, or pink eye. From the eyes… that is pretty kinky stuff. It shows up with headaches, fever, swollen lymph glands and maybe an ugly sore. Also a cause of infertility, it can present serious problems for a newborn baby. So, ladies, if you are playing around, you should consider being checked for the "clam" at least once a year.

NGU Sounds like the initials for a university with a great basketball team. Actually, it stands for nongonococcal urethritis, which in English, translates to "not the clap." It is a copycat condition which you can also pick up. Men don't have too much problem with it, a slight, thin discharge (known sometimes as the "little drip"). On the other hand, it can cause serious problems with the ladies interior plumbing.

Trichomoniasis This is a real nasty one, caused by a parasite. Yuk. It usually affects the gals much more than the guys, with possibly seven million cases a year. It is usually transmitted from women to men, but can also be passed from gal to gal by direct contact. She gets the worst of it— smelly, thick, yellowish discharge, higher susceptibility to HIV infection and even a possible chance of cervical cancer. Again, the "dudes" usually skate with little or no signs or effects.

Genital Warts (HPV) When guys are young they are invariably told that they will get warts on their hands if they masturbate. You could spot the guys who indulged the night before—checking their palms all day long. As guys get older they start realizing that a well-placed wart is supposed to be a big blessing. Well, it turns out that certain warts are not so good. More than a million persons a year, both men and women, are being blessed with new cases of this human papillomavirus, more commonly known as HPV and "genital warts." Although there is nothing funny about this abominable condition, it is difficult not to get tickled when you conjure up a picture of some guy with tiny cauliflowers growing all over the end of his wand. Not all infections have serious effects, but, once again, in the worst cases, women get screwed—a chance of cervical cancer lies in wait.

Pediculosis Pubis "Honest, I got it from a toilet seat." This time you can believe it—it's true. One of the most disgusting conditions known to man. Also identified as bloodsucking lice. No complete cure as yet. You can fight them with chemicals or freeze them with liquid nitrogen, but there is a good chance they will come back to visit another day. If these names don't ring a bell, you may have heard them referred to as the "Crabs." (Oh, yeah! Those guys.) Mean-looking, tiny little creatures, about the size of a pin-head. Yes, you can catch them from dirty toilet seats, bed spreads, sheets, hair brushes (remember their first-cousin, head lice) and, of course, body-to-body contact. There were unsubstantiated stories about pediculosi leaping across a room to get somebody. If you pick up a case of "crabs" you will likely be shunned by even your closest associates. You will learn how lepers used to feel. The crabs convey an image of ultimate sleaze, unkempt filthy scab-covered flesh and garbage-level living conditions. One suggested cure is to light your pubic hairs on fire and stab the little nits with an ice pick as they scurry away from the flaming bush. (Don't be unbelievably stupid and actually try this.)

HSV Genitalis Type II Feeling a bit squeamish? These are only the minor leagues. The major leagues are yet to come. The trendy plague of the seventies was HSV Genitalis Type II. You probably remember it as Herpes. Unfortunately, it is still alive and kicking—with an estimated forty-five million infected in the U.S.—and the number is growing. It sort of faded from the headlines to page 12 after being replaced by more horrible things. It is likely that you have had a form of herpes at some time in your life. You knew it as a "cold sore" on your lip—Herpes Simplex I. No big deal, but painful, as well as a pain in the ass. Somehow, that cold sore on the lips found its way to somebody's sexual parts and the rest is history. It was promoted to Type II, and found itself a home. Most of the time the viral invaders stay dormant. But, they get restless, and then they get active. Nasty devils. Their first appearance may be as simple pimples, but it does not take long for them to go into action. They turn into clear, sometimes crusty blisters (you don't need a road map to figure out where)... minimal pain for the guys, severe pain for the ladies—like open, mucous sores. Gory stuff. Often up to three weeks of endless ouch, several times a year. A pregnant woman can pass it on to her unsuspecting fetus as a potentially fatal brain infection. Thanks, Mom. Even though promising cures are on the horizon, Herpes is usually a lifetime companion.

Hepatitis B If you are like most folks, you thought of Hepatitis as something an unlucky geologist would pick up in the jungles of Guatemala after being chewed on by some nearly extinct species of multi-legged fanged insect. Within seconds the victim's eyeballs turn bright yellow, and his or her skin assumes an attractive hue of pastel chartreuse. Pure fiction. Welcome to the world of reality. Not only does Hepatitis B usually honor you with an eventual one-way trip to the undertaker, it is easier to pick up than AIDS, the clap, or just about any of the other dirty diseases that might infect the crotch area. And it is not really considered to be an STD. Sharing a tooth brush? Could be a big mistake. Kissing a bunch of strangers? Not smart. Unprotected sexual activity with a stranger or sharing a needle? Could be a sure bet for picking up this horrendous beauty. Not much in the way of symptoms at first. A little flu, maybe some jaundice, maybe not (that's the pastel chartreuse skin described above). Don't worry about a sure cure. There really isn't one. You might recover on your own, but don't count on it. There is a glimmer of somewhat positive news. If you plan to travel in the fast lane of life and fit the descriptive category of "high risk," there is a series of inoculations that may provide some form of immunity. Best of luck, friend.

Syphillis How about the grand daddy of all time? The "Old Joe," or more anciently, the "French Disease." There is some conjecture as to how far back this disease goes, with some experts claiming that there is reference to this disease in the Bible, and others claiming that Columbus's adventuresome crew brought back more than jewelry and trinkets from their travels to far away lands. Some biggies in history went to their maker with a torso full of spirochetes—such as Napoleon and Al Capone. Today, the "syph" is sort of holding its own—no big epidemic like the clap or chlamydia. The spooky thing about the symptoms is—no pain. Usually, the first thing that pops up is a weird looking painless sore, like a crater in the moon, with a crusty pus-filled center. This gruesome zit is called a "*chancre*," and usually—but not always—shows up near where the bug got transported from its donor. For the fairer sex, it may be hiding where it can't be seen and goes undetected. Nevertheless, you are contagious.

All you need at this point to clear things up is a few million units of penicillin. If not, and you wait long enough, the chancre goes away. Gone, but not forgotten! When it does come back, it comes disguised as an innocent rash. Doesn't even itch—maybe some hair loss, a little fever and mouth sores. If you go past this stage without treatment, you may well be history. You have reached the tertiary stage, and, at some time in the future, you might become a paralyzed zombie with a wasted heart and one foot in the grave.

Did you happen to notice a common trait found in all of these social scourges? Women are more likely to get serious, or even fatal, complications from almost all of them. So, gals—when you thought you were getting screwed ... guess what? You were absolutely right!

Got no protection? Forget that erection

This phrase should be the byword for all potential trysts. In this day and age there is absolutely no excuse for doing any sex-you-all activities without protection. In fact, any time Roger is out of his stall in intimate situations he should be covered. Besides the scourge of the above-mentioned STDs, an unwanted pregnancy can really mess up the everyday life of Charley Cooldude and Esther Easylay. Buying condoms now is as simple as picking up a quart of milk at the nearest convenience store. Things were not so "convenient" back in the "good old days." With few exceptions the only source was the pharmacist at the local drug store, who knew everyone in town's parents. Girls would never dream of trying to acquire them. It was up to the guys. The scenario usually went something like this:

Pharmacist ...   *can I help you, young man?*
Dude ...   *uh, yeah, I need some, uh, you know ...*
Pharmacist ...   *a prescription, maybe?*
Dude ... ...   *no, uh, ...a package of ... uh, you know ...* (squirm)
Pharmacist ...   *oh... O.K... what brand?*
Dude ...   *brand?... uh, uh ... don't matter ... uh ...* (squirm, sweat)
Pharmacist ...   *what size? ...*
Dude ... ... *uh... Size? Huh???* (<u>tremble</u>, squirm, sweat,)
Pharmacist ... ... *package of three, or a dozen?*
Dude ... ... *oh, oh, yeah ... uh, three* (audible sigh of relief)
Pharmacist ... *that will be a dollar* (smiling)

Fortunately, with such ready access today it is easy to avoid slip-ups and accidents. All of the effort you will have put into your program to increase sexual capacity and performance would be wasted with such a stupid mistake as picking up a case of some unnamed, incurable STD or creating an unexpected, unwanted surprise for all involved.

The Geriatric Factor

This section of the book was intended to educate the young and the restless about the dark side of uninhibited sexual activity. It seems now that a portion of the opposite end of the spectrum is in need of some facts of life. Menopause does not mean that the old ship is beached. Many of those horny senior citizens discussed earlier not only do it, they spread the joy by being sexually active with more than one partner. Such antiquarian activity, especially with the advent of "the little blue pill," has created a surge in senior sex and a disregard for the use of condoms. The result? Almost an epidemic of STDs in a nursing home complex in Southern Florida. It was reportedly so prolific that one local news reporter quoted a gynecologist as stating that she treated more cases of Herpes and HPV in this retirement community than she did in the City of Miami. One patient was in her eighties. You can probably take book that incidents like this are occurring everywhere, so no segment of the population is immune.

CONCLUSION

Fad diets come and go, and headlines of new exercise techniques appear every month on the covers of numerous magazines with promises of shedding excess flesh in a flash. Do they succeed? Obviously not, because diet attempts and corresponding exercise programs seem to last for the time it takes to drive, not walk, to the nearest fast food joint for the latest mega-monster-bigger-burger or gigantosoric super-meal. Special diets and exercise routines require tremendous effort, will power and desire to succeed. Failure followed by self-condemnation is almost a sure thing. Some semblance of a change in life style is a requisite. This book offers a simple laid-back approach without rules or schedules and no recriminations for lack of effort.

It should be self-evident that physical condition and vigorous sexual stamina go hand in hand. Some of the sex exercises may seem a bit odd or off the wall, but it doesn't cost anything to give them a try. If you took the effort to read the book, now all you have to do is put some of it to use. You might be quite pleased with the results.

ABOUT THE AUTHOR

Jerry Moore had considerable athletic experience, starting at age 12 when he won the Junior Olympics title at his housing project. Later he was league basketball player of the year in high school, and played freshman basketball at UCLA when John Wooden was head coach. Later he received an athletic scholarship to Louisiana State University and was on the track team with All American football player and Heisman Trophy winner Billy Cannon. While at LSU Moore set a school record in the pole vault and won the Southeastern Conference pole vault title.

He became interested in politics at an early age as student body president at Narbonne High School in Lomita, California. Years later he assisted in the incorporation of Lomita into a city, serving on the City council for ten years, two of them as Mayor. He retired as a fire Captain after 33 years with the Los Angeles County fire department. He has three children from his first marriage. In his second marriage, with two daughters, resided in Duncan, Oklahoma for several years where he and his wife gave ballroom dance lessons to about eighty of the local citizens. From there he moved to Sun Prairie, Wisconsin and was soon elected to the City Council, serving two years, one as Council President.

978-0-595-43370-4
0-595-43370-7

www.ingramcontent.com/pod-product-compliance
Lightning Source LLC
Chambersburg PA
CBHW030341290526
45785CB00004B/1557